BECOMING A THERAPIST

Becoming a Therapist

What Do I Say, and Why?

SUZANNE BENDER
EDWARD MESSNER

THE GUILFORD PRESS
New York   London

© 2003 The Guilford Press
A Division of Guilford Publications, Inc.
72 Spring Street, New York, NY 10012
www.guilford.com

Paperback edition 2004

Printed in the United States of America

This book is printed on acid-free paper.

Last digit is print number: 9 8 7 6 5 4

Library of Congress Cataloging-in-Publication Data

Bender, Suzanne
    Becoming a therapist : what do I say, and why? / by Suzanne Bender
and Edward Messner.
            p.   cm.
    ISBN 1-57230-804-4 (hardcover)   ISBN 1-57230-943-1 (paperback)
    1. Psychotherapy.   I. Messner, Edward.   II. Title.
RC480 .B359 2003
616.89′14—dc21
                                                        2002007092

To my mother and father, Meri and David Bender
—S. B.

To Marie Messner
—E. M.

About the Authors

Suzanne Bender, MD, is a Staff Psychiatrist, working with children and adolescents, at Massachusetts General Hospital (MGH) and Clinical Instructor in Psychiatry at Harvard Medical School. She received her medical degree from the University of California, San Francisco, and completed an adult psychiatry residency and child psychiatry fellowship at MGH. Dr. Bender received the MGH Psychiatry Department's Psychodynamic Writing Award in 1998. She also has a private practice, specializing in psychotherapy with adolescents and adults.

Edward Messner, MD, is a Senior Psychiatrist at Massachusetts General Hospital and an Associate Clinical Professor of Psychiatry at Harvard Medical School. He is a graduate of Harvard Medical School and, following an internship in San Francisco, attended the United States Air Force (USAF) School of Aviation Medicine. He was later awarded the USAF Commendation Ribbon for Meritorious Achievement as advisor to the Surgeon General of the Korean Air Force.

After his military service, Dr. Messner's psychiatric training consisted of 2 years of adult residency at the Boston Veterans Administration Hospital, 1 year of child fellowship at the Thom Clinic in Boston, and then 2 years as a clinical and research fellow at MGH. At the same time, he received training at the Boston Psychoanalytic Institute and was graduated as a certified psychoanalyst. During Dr. Messner's career in the MGH Psychiatry Department, which has been rated number one in the United States for 7 consecutive years, he has earned the Teacher of the Year award six times.

Prologue

I smiled at the empty chair, hoping my facial expression conveyed empathy and wisdom. In 15 minutes, my first psychotherapy patient would inhabit this seat, and as a solid believer in site-dependent learning, I hoped these final rehearsals would prepare me for the first moments of the upcoming session.

One more time, I ran through the details of my scripted introduction. I tried to assume an assortment of "empathic postures." I moved the box of tissues next to the unoccupied chair. I offered my outstretched hand to the empty space. "I'm Dr. Bender," I said in the most sensitive, professional tone I could muster. *Pause. Pause.* After the first hello, I was tongue-tied.

Before psychotherapy training, I never had trouble talking with patients. During a year of medical internship, communicating with the seriously ill seemed to be one of my strengths. Maybe my acute onset of wordlessness as a psychotherapy trainee was connected to my high personal expectations. I wanted to be very good. Well, to be honest, I wanted to be incredible. Instead, 1994 became my year to sweat as I intently listened to my first patients. I half expected (hoped? prayed?) that healing words would magically emerge from within me, heralding the first spontaneous psychiatric cure. You know, the patient enters the office in anguish and leaves 50 minutes later with renewed hope and faith in the human condition.

I majored in psychology in college and have some relatives who are therapists, so I hoped I would have a knack for this work. Needless to say, I was disappointed and had to learn the art of psychotherapy at the same painstakingly slow rate as everybody else.

During my first few years of training, I started my personal search for words: words that would calm, words that would firmly confront, and words that would comfort. Many of my supervisors gently teased me when I wrote down their advice verbatim for reference presession. Personally, I still think this approach makes perfect sense. In psychotherapy, words and sentences are the tools of intervention. A small modification in sentence structure changes a comment from judgmental to empathic. For example, the sentence "Your relationship with your husband seems complicated" is much less disparaging than the comment "You certainly have trouble dealing with your husband."

Despite this intensive preparation, I didn't coast through my first year as a psychotherapist. I endured patients who never showed for the first session and others who came to a few meetings and then vanished. I worried that I was inadvertently causing the recurrent flight reactions.

I fantasized about a sophisticated walkie-talkie system that would fit discreetly inside my ear and connect me to my supervisor's office. With this system, I could obtain the guidance I needed instantly during a difficult session. I could whisper into my hidden microphone while the patient blew her nose. "Dr. Messner, are you in? She's not talking at all. What should I do next?"

"10-4, Suzanne, why don't you ask her more about her relationship with her brother?"

"Gotcha. Thanks. Signing off for now. I'll keep you posted."

"What do you really *do* in there?" became my persistent question during my first years as a psychiatrist. I was taught almost nothing about the process of psychotherapy in medical school or internship. A mental review of psychotherapists in film wasn't helpful. Except for Judd Hirsch's portrayal of a sensitive therapist in the movie *Ordinary People* (and how many comforting comments can you glean from a few thoughtful scenes?), portrayals of sensitive, intelligent, and ethical therapists are hard to come by on the big screen. At best, therapists are featured as comic relief, quirky, and somewhat odd. At worst, they're sleeping with their patients or their patients' family members. In general, Hollywood provides a clear outline of what *not* to do.

While my beginning theory/technique courses and supervision provided some useful guidance, my questions emerged more quickly than they could be answered. From my novice's perspective, most books for the beginning therapist weren't very useful. One book advised me to create "a holding environment" for an agitated patient in crisis. Another stated that it was useful to "explore the resistance" for a patient who didn't want to talk. With only weeks of experience under my belt, I had no idea how to follow these recommendations.

To make matters worse, the patients in these texts were entirely too well behaved. They came on time; they understood complex interpretations; and they talked openly about their transference to the therapist. I didn't feel I could apply the interventions created for such extraordinarily sophisticated exemplars to my practice of ordinary patients without prior psychotherapy experience. Meanwhile, my clinic was growing, and I found myself embroiled in many complex clinical situations. What I needed were explicit directions telling me what to do, what to say, and why.

The roots of *Becoming a Therapist: What Do I Say, and Why?* took hold during an innocent conversation at the Massachusetts General Hospital (MGH) cafeteria with Dr. Edward Messner, a primary mentor and teacher at MGH with a special ability to explain arcane psychotherapeutic concepts in a clear and concise manner. He has won numerous Teacher of the Year awards, most recently in 1999. On a whim, I told Dr. Messner of my hope to write a book someday that would explain how to practice psychotherapy to the interested but confused beginner. I figured I'd be able to advise others once I had more experience, maybe when I was about 50. Instead of waiting 20 years, Dr. Messner proposed we write the book together—now. For me, it was one of those "aha" moments: Our collaboration was the perfect way to organize a book geared for the novice psychotherapist. I am still in touch with all the gnawing questions that bother a beginner, and Dr. Messner can explain what to do clearly and concisely, based on more than 40 years of clinical experience.

Although our original intention was to produce an instructive book for clinicians only, I was delighted when a number of friends, ranging from writers to lawyers, were intrigued by our project. It turns out that psychotherapists aren't the only ones with questions about psychotherapy. People are curious about what goes on during talking treatment, including how therapists think or feel, and what they say—and why. As we revised our text, we have kept our nontherapist readers in mind. We have included a glossary to define the technical terms that we could not reasonably avoid. The book still "talks" directly to the beginning clinician, but the information should be accessible to nontherapists as well.

The text before you represents our combined judgment. Common predicaments faced by the beginning psychotherapist will be presented in my voice while explanations and guidance will be presented in the plural, as our collaborative effort. Innumerable hours of supervision, with colleagues and mentors, also helped me to formulate my questions and to find my own answers. We gratefully recognize these clinicians in the acknowledgments.

We don't pretend to have the answers to every situation that you will encounter with your patients; the process of psychotherapy is as complex and variable as the patients and the therapists who engage in it. Instead, we hope that the outlined concepts and approaches will guide you as you develop your own voice. This book will lead you through the basics of psychotherapy: how to start seeing a patient, how to continue through the inevitable difficulties inherent in the process, how to understand what you are doing and why, and finally, how to terminate a treatment. Our greatest hope is that this book will provide for you what I was looking for just a few years ago.

List of Dialogues

I. The Consultation

Chapter 1. First Contact

Chapter 2. The First Moments

Chapter 3. Initiating an Alliance and Assessing Safety

Chapter 16. Transference and Countertransference

Chapter 17. Termination

Contents

Introduction

Becoming a psychotherapist is an unusual experience. Some of my teachers have compared psychotherapy to an impromptu dance between two partners. You can plan the first "hello" and "thank you" at the end of the set, but what happens between the greetings is unpredictable. However, if you are familiar with some basic and common dance steps, you will have an easier time improvising with a new partner. Psychotherapy is similar. Advanced therapists have an expansive repertoire of "steps" at their disposal. They are comfortable dealing with the basics in psychotherapy, so they can tailor each treatment to meet the unique needs of a patient.

This book's purpose is to teach you the basic steps one needs to know fluently to practice psychotherapy. It is not a cookbook of what to say and when, but a guidebook to help the beginner understand and resolve common clinical dilemmas. We outline some common predicaments that emerge in many treatments and then evaluate a variety of responses.

As physicians, we refer to the person seeking therapy as a patient, but some therapists may prefer mentally to substitute the term "client." Throughout the book, we have tried to avoid jargon so the text can be understood by a wide range of readers, including clinicians, patients, potential patients, and inquisitive laypersons.

THE BASICS

What is psychotherapy suppposed to do? Psychotherapy can help patients cope with traumas, crises, losses, and developmental changes. It can enable people to bring out the best in themselves by recognizing and then discarding ineffective approaches to life's challenges and by discovering talents, capacities, and strengths that were previously buried. The psychotherapeutic relationship itself is involved in the healing process. It can provide a model for mature and empathic interactions and can foster the development of problem-solving skills in emotionally laden situations. By removing the obstacles to personal maturation, psychotherapy can help a patient discover inner complexity, richness, beauty, and worth.

For psychotherapy to occur, the patient must make it to the therapist's office. This is no little achievement. By calling for an appointment, the patient is acknowledging that she has an emotional conflict or difficulty that has not improved despite her best efforts. Often, the trip to the therapist is the patient's last resort. Since psychotherapy is poorly understood by many people, it is often shunned and considered only after other remedies (i.e., exercise, relaxation, friendly advice, vitamin supplements, etc.) have failed.

Interestingly, as a treatment evolves, it may focus on a conflict very different from the one that first brought the patient to the office. For example, a patient may start therapy complaining about her self-centered partner who is unresponsive to her many thoughtful gestures. Although the beginning of treatment may concentrate on the patient's relationship, eventually the focus may shift. Why is the patient drawn to such an unfulfilling partner in the first place? After some discussion of present and past difficulties, it may become clear that the patient has a maladaptive behavior pattern, pulling her toward self-absorbed companions.

Here's where the work in psychotherapy becomes difficult. If it were easy to act differently or to feel better, the patient wouldn't need therapy in the first place. Underneath an emotional conflict that doesn't seem to make sense (e.g., why is this person always attracted to unsupportive partners?) there may lurk multiple intrapsychic forces that oppose more adaptive behaviors. These forces are powerful. They have to be; they've repeatedly interfered with the patient's ability to act in a way that would promote her own happiness or productivity.

As therapists, it is our duty and responsibility to recognize these forces, to respect them, and then to learn about them in careful detail. As looking at one's emotional blemishes isn't easy, the treatment must explore the patient's difficulties in a nonpejorative and compassionate manner. The goal of therapy is to understand the powerful grip of these patterns of belief and emotion. They wouldn't exist unless they had been useful once, but by the time a person finds her way to therapy, they tend to be obsolete and harmful.

When the patient is able to understand and to integrate both the thinking and feeling parts of her unconscious motivations, emotional growth and change is possible. Learning this information unaccompanied by the emotions that travel with it or feeling hurt and angry without grasping its source isn't therapeutic. For emotional change to occur, both the feelings and thoughts involved in a conflict need to be understood. Only then can the patient recognize that she has choices; before this realization, her maladaptive behavior had appeared to be automatic and to be the only option available. As treatment progesses, the patient can choose more adaptive courses, but she often needs additional help with this aspect of her personal development.

Underlying any treatment strategy is our recognition that many inner conflicts, fears, and motivations originate outside the conscious awareness of the patient. The powerful influences of early experience need to be understood for the patient to improve. An understanding of psychodynamic therapy can inform any type of treatment, especially when complications such as noncompliance or self-defeating behaviors arise.

Specialized therapies also exist. Cognitive-behavioral therapy focuses predominately on beliefs, attitudes, and actions. Psychopharmacological treatment uses medication to change the patient's neurochemical milieu.

This book includes elements of all these approaches. We believe the well-prepared therapist needs to have a variety of potential interventions available in her repertoire. For this reason, our approach could be called integrative.

We hope the reader will learn how to cultivate and to preserve a therapeutic environment that will allow any appropriate type of therapy to flourish. Our intention is to help the reader provide the treatment that is most beneficial to the patient, one that is shaped to her specific needs.

In order to illustrate, word for word, how to approach many basic issues that commonly emerge in a psychodynamic psychotherapy, Dr. Messner and I invented our virtual patient, Sallie Gane, a 21-year-old college junior. With Sallie Gane, it's possible for the reader to be the fly on the wall, listening in to Sallie's psychotherapy with me, her hypothetical therapist. Her story will unfold over time, just as it would in a typical treatment. Notations describing Sallie's tone of voice, facial expressions, gestures, and postures will describe some of her nonverbal communications. Similar notations for the therapist are also included, as a therapist's body language complements any spoken word and is a vital part of any effective treatment.

As I experience typical psychotherapeutic dilemmas in my interactions with Sallie, the book will illustrate a variety of possible responses. The titles of the dialogues inform the reader whether the example is an illustration of a clinically effective strategy or is one worth avoiding. The

List of Dialogues in the front matter of the book shows the title of each dialogue in this volume so that the inquiring psychotherapist can quickly search for specific clinical guidance.

Sallie's treatment illustrates the basics of therapy in a cohesive framework, but her psychological conflicts are more simple than those found in typical clinic patients. She is not struggling with economic hardship; she doesn't currently abuse substances; her health is intact; and she is not a victim of physical, sexual, or emotional abuse. For teaching purposes, the therapy centered on a key conflict with her mother and her brother. While some treatments may spend more time focusing on the relationship with one parent, it would be very unusual for the focus to be this exclusive, as most patients have been influenced by numerous people, including both parents. Still, we hope the strategies and words we offer in response to Sallie's difficulties will be transferable to psychotherapies with your patients.

Since Sallie Gane, the patient we will discuss in most detail, is female, we have employed feminine pronouns for general usage. With few exceptions, "she" should be read to mean "she or he" and "her" should be read to mean "her or his."

The first part of the book, titled *The Consultation*, outlines how to approach the first few sessions with a new patient. It begins with the first phone call to set up an appointment and ends with an explanation of psychotherapy for a patient unfamiliar with the process.

The second part of the book, titled *Frame and Variations*, explains how talking with a therapist is different from talking to a friend. This section explains the importance of the ground rules of the therapy (such as starting and ending at a particular time) that may seem especially arbitrary or capricious to the beginning clinician. This section also illustrates how to handle situations in which the boundaries of treatment are violated.

Part III, *Chemistry*, focuses on harmful and helpful drugs relevant to psychotherapeutic practice. Chapter 12 presents ways to recognize and to treat patients with substance abuse problems. Chapter 13 offers suggestions how to coordinate psychotropic medication treatment with psychotherapy.

The last part of the book, titled *Therapeutic Dilemmas*, discusses how to approach more complex issues that may emerge within a therapy, such as dreams, interpretations, and transference. Overall, this section focuses on the intricate process of therapy, rather than the basic rules that create the treatment's foundation.

Throughout the book, additional ficitious patients are introduced to discuss topics not included in Sallie's treatment. Candice Jones, a patient who has some trouble differentiating what is real from what is fantasy when she is under stress, appears intermittently in multiple chapters (Chapters 5, 11, 16, and 17), illustrating a specialized treatment approach for patients with this type of difficulty. Anthony Lee in Chapter 12 struggles with alcohol abuse. His story describes how the therapist's strategy must change when dealing with a patient who is actively abusing substances. Chapter 13 introduces another patient, Elaine Barber, to highlight the therapeutic issues that emerge when treating a patient with psychotherapy and psychotropic medications. We have also used references to actual patients to supplement the dialogues. In these cases, multiple clinical details have been changed to make the patient unrecognizable.

Sallie is only one person with one cultural history. Since cultures and ethnic traditions vary widely within the United States (e.g., the cultures of the Los Angeles African American, Asian, Latino, or Jewish communities are much different from those of their counterparts in New York City), there is no way to know the details of every potential subculture of every patient you will treat. Therefore, we advocate a sensitivity and interest in cultural, religious, ethnic, socioeconomic, gender, and sexuality issues that highlight the uniqueness of each patient's experience.

In case you want to learn more about a particular topic, we have included a list of key words and technical terminology at the end of each chapter that can guide a literature search on the Internet. Psychological terms used in the text are defined in the Glossary.

So there you have it. Read on, and the therapy with Sallie begins, starting with her first message on my answering machine. How should I respond to her phone call? This is the type of question that used to plague me. Our hope is that this text will provide answers to these types of basic questions, explaining the "what," "why," and, most crucial for the beginner, the "how" of psychotherapy.

Part I
The Consultation

1

First Contact

The patient's initial phone call may be a challenge for the novice therapist. It is the first opportunity to set the stage for future treatment. Answering this call should be approached with the patient's privacy and concerns in mind.

THE PHONE CALL

"Hi, my name is Sally Gane and my primary care doctor gave me your number. I think I am interested in therapy. Could you call me back? My number is 555-2121."

Before I pick up the phone to return Sally's call, I want to acknowledge how anxious I felt with my first psychotherapy referral. It was difficult to embrace a professional identity that had been in place only 48 hours. I reacted with an acute bout of indigestion.

My friends with similar psychosomatic tendencies reported feeling flushed and then concerned that they may have suddenly acquired high blood pressure. Some colleagues coped by skimming large psychotherapy texts during occasional spare moments between patient care and seminars. One classmate seemed unnaturally calm and overconfident, and spouted comments like "Psychotherapy is all intuition anyway. I trust my instincts, so I know I am ready to treat just about anybody."

Basically, all of these reactions demonstrate the varied ways of managing the intense and normal anxiety that most psychotherapy trainees experience. Your supervisors probably had similar worries when they began training, but they may have successfully submerged these memories as they gained expertise. On the bright side, anxiety can be advantageous when it's motivating but not overwhelming. Our recommendation is to acknowledge the fact that you are worried and to share your experience with sensitive colleagues for support. Anxiety usually increases if you fight the fact that you have it in the first place.

A psychotherapy trainee who can acknowledge that she has a lot to learn is in the best position to help her patients. The process of psychotherapy is all about "not knowing" and having the patient teach you about her experience. Provided that you listen attentively to her replies, the more questions you ask your patient, the more the two of you will learn together. The more questions you ask your supervisor, the more you will learn about the case you are discussing. A grandiose "I-know-everything" or "Here's-the-answer" approach does not serve your patients well, especially if you hesitate to seek the guidance you will undoubtably need.

When I started learning psychotherapy, I felt guilty that my patients would be stuck with me as their therapist, rather than a more experienced clinician in the community. Many of my friends shared my concern. As Dr. Messner taught us in the first days of residency, beginnning therapists have something very special to offer. A quote: "The first patients of a psychotherapy trainee are lucky." Yes, lucky.

Under a trainee's care, patients will receive enthusiastic, caring, and attentive treatment from an interested and compassionate psychotherapist. Via supervision, the patient will also benefit from clinical expertise. This combination can provide for a thoughtful and helpful treatment that may have advantages over a treatment received in the community where energy, idealism, and optimism may have subsided. I've even heard patients brag about being their therapist's first patient and about how proud they were to be in this unique position.

Although it may seem obvious to some, we want to share a common and effective coping mechanism that can alleviate first-session jitters. Whatever your current state during the consultation with a new patient, the patient is bound to be the more anxious individual in the room. She is the one who has decided to confide in a stranger because of persistent emotional difficulties. Setting up the first appointment may have been a formidable task that took weeks to months. Whenever a psychotherapy becomes complicated or anxiety-provoking for the therapist, it can revitalize compassion and calm to remember how the patient must feel.

For the skeptics in the audience, we want to review why we are spending a chapter discussing how to answer a phone message, a seemingly uncomplicated event. A therapist's response to a phone message from a potential psychotherapy patient counts as the first clinical interaction. It is the therapist's first opportunity to demonstrate the unique attributes of the therapeutic relationship. The therapist's focus is on the patient, but the interaction is professional with specific and strict limitations. With this in mind, even the words the therapist chooses to leave on Sally's answering machine are relevant in setting the stage and tone for a potential therapeutic relationship and for future communications.

So, how to respond?

I don't know the details of Sally's living situation. She may live alone, or she may share an answering machine with her best friend, a houseful of people, or even her parents. I also don't know whether Sally has shared her decision to start psychotherapy with her roommates, whoever they may be. These circumstances necessitate leaving a relatively discreet message on her answering machine if she is not home.

To protect privacy, I use words that do not scream "psychotherapy" when returning a message. The upcoming session can be referred to as an "appointment" or "meeting." Since I have not met Sally yet, I may choose to address her in a more formal manner—"Sally Gane" or "Ms. Sally Gane."

I feel most comfortable referring to myself in a first phone message as Suzanne Bender, not Dr. Suzanne Bender. Other clinicians disagree with this approach, stating that it is important to use one's professional title consistently. There are pros and cons to both points of view. On the one hand, if I address my future patient in a more formal manner on the phone, it may be more consistent to use my title as well. Yet if I am leaving a message, I have no way of knowing who might hear it. A phone message from a doctor is bound to fuel questions from housemates. A bland message from an unidentified person (Suzanne Bender, instead of Dr. Suzanne Bender) is less likely to spur curiosity. Personally, I err on the side of protecting the patient's privacy until I know more about the patient's living situation.

While returning a message may seem like a simple communication, some messages facilitate future interactions better than others. Here's an example of a message that could lead to a mishap:

EXAMPLE 1.1

The therapist's vague phone message in response to the patient's first call

THERAPIST: Hello, this is Suzanne Bender returning a message from Ms. Sally Gane. You can call me at my pager, 555-0001, or I'll call back tonight so we can set up a meeting time.

While this message seems relatively straightforward, its vague directions set the stage for future "phone tag." First, I don't clarify when I'll be available to answer pages (or when I will be in the office and able to answer the phone) without delay. The patient may page me while I'm commuting home and therefore unable to return the call for many minutes. By the time I answer the call, I may have to continue my dialogue with the answering machine. I'm then left in the uncomfortable position of chasing my new patient to set up a meeting time.

Some possible solutions:

First, I try to answer initial phone calls in the early evening hours, when I am more likely to contact the potential patient in person. If it is still difficult to get in touch with the patient, the following message is an effective option.

EXAMPLE 1.2

The therapist's clear phone message in response to the patient's first call

THERAPIST: Hello, this is Suzanne Bender calling for Sally Gane. I received your message. To reach me, you can page me tomorrow between the hours of 9:00 and 1:00. My pager number is 555-0001. At these times, I am able to answer fairly quickly. If we are unable to connect today or tomorrow, please leave me a message with some good times that I can reach you.

By stating the times I can promptly answer a page (or phone call), I might avoid a call during off hours. Also, once I ask Sally to list times she will be available, she becomes responsible for getting in touch with me, rather than vice versa.

So, then, the first conversation occurs.

EXAMPLE 1.3

The first phone conversation: In her excitement, the therapist agrees to meet at an inopportune time

THERAPIST: Hi, is this Ms. Sally Gane?

SALLY GANE: Yes.

THERAPIST: Hi, this is Dr. Suzanne Bender; I got your message.

SALLY: Oh, hi. I got your name from Dr. Newman, my doctor at school.

THERAPIST: You mentioned in your message that you might be interested in therapy. Can you tell me a little bit about what you are looking for?

SALLY: Umm, well, I don't know. . . . Do you do therapy?

THERAPIST: I do. I have my schedule book open. Would you like to set up a time to meet?

SALLY: Okay.

THERAPIST: What days are possible for you?

SALLY: Well, I am working part time and going to school, so my schedule is a bit tight. But I could meet at Tuesday at 7:00 P.M. or Friday at 6:00 P.M.?

THERAPIST: (*Feels stomach sink at thought of meeting so late in the day, but doesn't know what else to do but to agree.*) Okay, I think Tuesday at 7:00 would be fine.

SCHEDULING

With my first psychotherapy patients, I agreed to almost any meeting time, no matter how awful, because I didn't want to lose the potential patient by being less accessible. With more experience, my strategy changed. Now, before I return a call to set up a first appointment, I outline the hours I have available for new patients. During the initial phone call, I only offer these session times, and avoid scheduling people during protected times that feel too late or too early.

While the time of the first consultation does not commit the therapist to that time for future therapy, the patient might develop that expectation. If Friday evening at 6:00 is a one-time event, the therapist needs to review her time restrictions when discussing future contacts.

During my first year as a therapist, I spent my Wednesday mornings commuting at an ungodly hour to meet one patient at 6:30 A.M. At first, I really didn't mind. I was so excited to have any patient interested in working with me. We started meeting during the summer when the sun had already risen before my 30-minute commute. My patient's attendance was perfect; and the session with him was the highlight of my day.

By December, I was no longer so excited by our arrangement. The absurdity of the schedule hit home the day I spent 15 minutes inching down an icy hill toward my subway stop before sunrise. Then my patient didn't show up. When I called to find out what had happened, he said it was too cold to come to such an early appointment.

This missed session was just the first of his many wintertime no-shows. I tried to reschedule his weekly time, but he insisted that this was the only hour he could meet with me during the entire week. I was caught in a frequent beginner's quandary: I was more invested in his therapy than he was, and I didn't feel comfortable setting limits regarding the meeting time. (Words I could have used: "Unfortunately, I can no longer continue meeting at 6:30 A.M. Let's look at our schedules together and come up with a solution.") Meanwhile, my patient continued to attend only every second or third session and I continued to spend Wednesday mornings in a fury. Ultimately, the therapy suffered. I was not as sensitive or engaged as I might have been. How could I be when I was fuming inside?

I hope to protect you from this type of mistake. Safeguarding your own time is a crucial part of being an effective therapist. Meeting the patient's needs with an awkward meeting time may eventually backfire when the therapy suffers due to your increasing resentment.

Patients who work are ordinarily available mornings and evenings. To make room for these patients and simultaneously to heed your own needs, you can schedule patients with full work schedules at early or late hours, depending on your own working style. Before I had my first child, I preferred to start working early in the morning, but now, as a working mother, I have one evening clinic a week for my hard-to-schedule patients.

When I end up in a scheduling nightmare that I didn't anticipate and don't want to tolerate, I've tried to view the situation as an educational experience. I use supervision to examine what made it so difficult to set limits. Once the dilemma is discussed and understood, my irate feelings are dispelled, and I can consider how I can sensitively broach a schedule change with the patient.

Let's play back the first phone conversation, illustrating how I could protect my schedule by offering a number of reasonable appointment times.

EXAMPLE 1.4

The first phone conversation: The therapist sets up a viable appointment time

THERAPIST: Hi, is this Ms. Sally Gane?

SALLY: Yes.

THERAPIST: Hi, this is Dr. Suzanne Bender; I got your message.

SALLY: Oh, hi. I got your name from Dr. Newman, my doctor at school.

THERAPIST: You mentioned in your message that you might be interested in therapy. Can you tell me a little bit about what you are looking for?

SALLY: Umm, well, I don't know. . . . Do you do therapy?

THERAPIST: Yes. I would be glad to meet with you for a consultation. I have my schedule book open. Would you like to set up a time to meet?

SALLY: Okay.

THERAPIST: What days are possible for you?

SALLY: Well, I am working part-time and going to school, so my schedule is a bit tight. But I could meet at Tuesday at 7:00 P.M. or Friday at 6:00 P.M.?

THERAPIST: I don't have either of those times available. My latest time available during the week is 6:00 P.M. on Tuesday, but I have some morning times available as well as some lunch hours. What about 8:00 A.M. on Thursday?

SALLY: Oh, I can't do that. I do have Monday afternoons open.

THERAPIST: What about this Monday, July 6th, at 2:00 P.M.?

SALLY: Oh, I actually can do that.

THERAPIST: Good. I'm glad we found a time. Would you like to discuss my fee now, or during the first visit?

SALLY: Um, can we discuss it during the meeting? Is that okay?

THERAPIST: Sure. Now let me give you directions to my office.

Example 1.4 also illustrates how I bring up my fee during the first phone call. The question ("Would you like to discuss my fee now, or during the first visit?") broaches the topic of money in a respectful yet open manner. An alternative approach would be to ask "Do you have health insurance?" and then discuss whether the insurance covered your services.

Since most novice psychotherapists train in a clinic where the administrative staff handles the billing, I have not included an in-depth discussion of financial and insurance issues in this chapter. I did need to know how to discuss fees and payments once I started to see private patients. We review how to set a fee and how to bill patients and/or insurance companies in more detail in Chapter 8.

As my phone call with Sally draws to a close, it is useful to obtain some basic information.

THERAPIST: Before we stop for now, for my records, may I have the correct spelling of your name and your address?

SALLY: Oh, yes. I spell my first name with an "ie"—so it is "S-a-l-l-i-e."
My last name is Gane, G-a-n-e. My address is 1111 Central Street
in Boston.

THERAPIST: What is the zip code?

SALLY: Um, it is 02114.

Spelling a patient's name correctly conveys respect and consideration.
I ask for this information during the consultation because it may become
awkward to insert this simple question into an ongoing treatment. I try
never to assume how to spell a patient's name since I've been wrong before.
Even simple names may have unusual spellings, as in this case, as Sallie
spells her name with an "ie" rather than the traditional "y."

I never know when I might need a patient's address during a therapy, so I also collect this information in the first phone call or during the
first meeting. In a psychiatric emergency, an address can be life saving. If
Sallie leaves treatment abruptly, I might need to send her a letter or bill
by mail. Problems in confidentiality can also be avoided by having a pre-
cise address. My use of the phrase "for my records" emphasizes the professional nature of the contract and reinforces the privacy that is protected in therapy.

Sallie may have some questions before the conversation ends.

SALLIE: Um, I was just wondering, before we meet, what is your psychological orientation?

THERAPIST: What do you mean?

SALLIE: Well, I am taking a psychology course and they are discussing
self psychology versus cognitive-behavioral psychology versus a
psychoanalytic approach to therapy. What's your approach?

THERAPIST: Well, I use an eclectic approach that integrates teachings
from many of the schools but emphasizes psychodyamic psychotherapy.

SALLIE: What about cognitive-behavioral techniques?

THERAPIST: Can you tell me what you are looking for?

SALLIE: I don't know really. I just want to know more about what to expect.

THERAPIST: I do incorporate some cognitive-behavioral therapy strategies into treatment, but rather than discussing this now, I would like
to give these questions the time they deserve. I hope we can talk
more about them when we meet, and you can let me know your
concerns or preferences.

SALLIE: Okay, I'll see you then.

THERAPIST: I look forward to meeting you on Monday, the 6th, at 2:00.

When setting up a first meeting, I try to keep the conversation simple and clear by validating the patient's concerns but avoiding a lengthy discussion that could be prone to misunderstandings.

It isn't unusual for a patient to express concerns about the therapeutic process as early as the first phone call. Sometimes these questions may reflect the patient's ambivalence regarding treatment. If she expresses significant hesitation about psychodynamic psychotherapy or a definite preference for another genre of treatment, I may provide alternative referral options. (Please see Chapter 6 for details on some of the more common options that are available for psychological treatment.)

FRAMING THE FIRST VISITS AS A CONSULTATION

We view the first few sessions with a patient as a consultation, not the beginning of treatment. The consultation consists of a few meetings during which I will obtain a history, make a diagnosis, and recommend a treatment plan. The package does not include a guarantee that I will become the patient's individual psychotherapist. In fact, until the consultation is complete, I cannot assume that individual psychotherapy is even the treatment of choice.

Framing the meeting as the first session of a consultation has a number of advantages. Before committing to treatment, the patient can test whether she feels comfortable talking to me, and I can ascertain whether I feel capable of treating her. Both of us are given the freedom to view the first meeting as an introduction without an obligation to continue.

The consultation approach allows each person to see whether the two individuals are a "good match," a term commonly used in psychological circles. A "good match" means that the patient feels understood and willing to work with the clinician, and the clinician feels hopeful about her ability to work with the patient effectively.

Now and then, a patient may feel misunderstood by a therapist from the moment she steps into the office. Sometimes the clinician can turn this situation to therapeutic advantage by understanding why the patient is so uncomfortable (see Chapter 16). However, bad matches also exist. Sometimes the patient and therapist just don't "click." Certain people may work together more easily, depending on whether the patient is searching for a therapist with a style similar to or different than her own. A shy, withdrawn woman may find a charismatic and interactive male therapist either overwhelming or energizing. Alternatively, a dramatic person may prefer a therapist with a similar disposition, or one with a more low-key, soft-spoken approach.

I've found it's best to explain the consultation process very early on to reduce the likelihood of future misunderstanding. Some therapists choose to review this information over the phone while setting up the the first appointment so the arrangement is clear before the patient enters the office. In Sallie's treatment, I mention that the initial meeting is a consultation during our phone conversation, and explain the process in detail during our first session, in Chapters 2 and 3. As you meet many different individuals and start many different therapies, it can be helpful to try out multiple approaches in order to weigh the pros and cons of each, first-hand.

Key words: confidentiality, consultation, evaluation, help seeking, identifying information, privacy, psychiatric evaluation, psychotherapy, psychotherapy scheduling

2

The First Moments

First impressions during the the initial visit of a psychotherapeutic consultation are important. The therapist should greet the new patient in a manner that will protect her confidentiality. The session begins with an open question that facilitates conversation.

INTRODUCTIONS

Sallie Gane checks herself into the clinic and sits down in the public waiting area. She is 20 minutes early. She nervously picks up a news magazine and flips through it quickly. I start my internal countdown: 10 minutes to 2:00 P.M., 5 minutes to 2:00. . . .

I felt more like a fraud than a clinician with my first patients. I agonized over the fact that I couldn't prepare beforehand for the first meetings. I could orchestrate my greeting, but it was impossible to choreograph the rest of the session before hearing what the patient had to say. As a novice, I reviewed my first session plan with Dr. Messner.

To be honest, I hadn't expected to have such a long discussion with him about it. "Dr. Messner," I'd started, "I'll call out my patient's name in the waiting room, and we'll walk into the office together, but then what do I do?" He paused and didn't answer my question right away. Instead, we discussed whether my current plan of action adequately protected my patient's confidentiality. I hadn't considered that privacy was a therapeutic issue before the patient even entered the office.

As Dr. Messner explained, protecting a patient's confidentiality must be a priority. By calling my patient's name in a common waiting area, I would have failed to safeguard her identity. For psychotherapy to be successful, the therapist must earn the patient's trust by respecting and protecting her privacy from the moment that the treatment begins.

Dr. Messner knew of a priest who had been struggling with his vow of celibacy and had come to psychotherapy for help in clarifying his future role in the church. The priest was wearing layman's clothes and was holding hands with a woman while he waited for his appointment. His psychotherapist entered the public waiting room and greeted him with "Hello, Father." The low-level buzz in the waiting room ceased; people stared and whispered. The therapist's seemingly innocent greeting was embarrassing at best, humiliating at worst: not the best way to instill trust in a new relationship.

To avoid making a similar mistake when I met my patient, Dr. Messner recommended that I identify myself without calling out her name. With this strategy, I could protect her identity just in case she was indirectly connected with someone in the waiting area. Her decision to seek psychiatric consultation would remain private. (For more discussion of confidentiality, please see Chapter 11.)

EXAMPLE 2.1

A method of introduction that preserves the patient's confidentiality

Sallie Gane now waits expectantly in the waiting room. There are four other people waiting for other clinicians.

I ask the secretary who checked her in to point her out to me. I approach her cautiously since I have not confirmed that she is my new patient.

THERAPIST: Excuse me, who are you waiting to see?

SALLIE: Dr. Bender?

THERAPIST: Hello, I'm Dr. Bender. Let me show you to my office.

SALLIE: Thanks. I'm Sallie.

If Sallie didn't offer her name spontaneously after my introduction, I could confirm her identity in the office with a prompt: "And your name is . . . " or "I'm sorry, I didn't catch your name. . . . "

On first impression, I thought Example 2.1 seemed like introduction gymnastics. I didn't feel grateful for Dr. Messner's clear and sensitive explanation. In fact, I felt resentful of the advice that felt too intricate and restrictive. I checked with a few other supervisors to see whether they agreed with his approach. Interestingly, they were all completely unanimous on this issue. Privacy first . . . and always, they said.

I still felt upset. With these new rules, I felt bound in a social strait-jacket. I felt sure that Sallie would think my specially concocted intro-duction was extremely strange. I also imagined many awkward moments standing by a full waiting room, asking if anyone was here to see me and getting no response. It didn't feel natural to act in such a ritualistic man-ner. One other worry: if I couldn't even figure out how to say hello with-out supervision, what damage might I do in an entire session? It took a few deep breaths and some cathartic complaining sessions with my fel-low trainees before I was ready to accept this unfamiliar approach.

It helped to think about learning psychotherapy as similar to learn-ing a new sport. When you start to play a new game, such as basketball, it initially feels very strange to dribble and shoot the ball. The moves don't feel natural, because they aren't, but they are necessary in order to play the game well. The moves in psychotherapy, such as the introduc-tion to a patient, involve using everyday language in unique ways. Ini-tially these procedures feel constraining and maybe even a bit bizarre, but, within the realm of psychotherapy, they are appropriate.

I followed Dr. Messner's advice and was surprised that my real pa-tients didn't react to my new greeting with raised eyebrows and "Who are you?" looks. In fact, I have a definite sense that certain treatments would have been in trouble if I hadn't carefully protected patient confi-dentiality from the first moment. Over time, what initally felt like an odd greeting ritual began to feel natural and normal. Many interventions in psychotherapy are like this, uncomfortable and stiff at first, but useful and easier with time.

Sallie Gane stands up. I smile and she smiles back. She extends her hand. Should I take it?

Some very traditional psychotherapists question whether even mini-mal physical contact, such as an introductory handshake, is appropriate between therapist and patient. Because a handshake is such an accepted greeting in American culture, we think avoiding a handshake may feel rejecting. The handshake will also give you nonverbal information. Does the patient extend her hand comfortably, or is she more cautious? Is her grip firm or loose? An interesting note: As therapy does try to minimize all types of physical contact, this may be the last time you touch your pa-tient, unless you shake her hand good-bye at the end of the treatment.

Would I extend my hand first? While I don't think a correct answer exists, I've personally decided not to initiate handshakes. During these first moments, I don't know anything about my new patient. She may be avoiding a handshake because of underlying paranoia or a thought dis-order. Setting the stage for future therapy interactions, I follow the pa-tient's lead, even with the basic hello.

I lead Sallie into my office. She moves toward the chair that I usually sit in; my bookbag clearly propped against the chair's leg. What should I do?

After I received detailed and unexpected advice about how to choreograph introductions, I worried about other unanticipated clinical situations. Maybe there was a special rule that the patient sits in the office chair she prefers no matter what the therapist's previous plans. Luckily, clinical situations that don't involve confidentiality are best approached with straightforward common sense. In this case, as the therapist, it is important that *you* feel comfortable in *your* chair with easy access to your desk, telephone, notepad, or other items. If I were stuck in the situation just outlined, I could point to the appropriate chair and redirect Sallie with a quick comment: "Could you take this chair, please?" or "Please sit here."

SETTING UP THE OFFICE

Psychotherapists have minimal overhead. To practice this type of treatment, all I really need is four walls, a couple of chairs, and a phone.

Therapists arrange the chairs in their office at various distances, depending on their own culture and style. If the patient and I might kick each other's feet by accident, we're too close. Depending on the population I am working with, I might set up the room so that I am closer to the door, allowing for a quick exit in case a patient becomes physically threatening. I hope I never have to escape from my office, but in case of an emergency, this setup would facilitate an easy departure.

Talking across a desk can be very formal and not conducive to intimate conversation; my patient may feel like an employee reporting to her superior. I can use the desk to my advantage if the patient sits at the end of the desk, and I talk to her across the desk's corner. This set up is relaxed and may feel less threatening than sitting face to face across open space.

In contrast to many other health professionals who display pictures of their families at their desks, psychotherapists tend to avoid placing personal photos in public view. Personal mementos draw attention away from the patient's intimate concerns and may make it more difficult for the patient to focus on her own experience and to talk about issues that may be shaming or painful. Family pictures also pique a patient's curiosity, communicating an inconsistent message when the therapist refuses to share further personal information.

Interestingly, many psychotherapists practice psychotherapy in a home office, but do not decorate the professional space with personal items. Nevertheless, interested patients will pay detailed attention to the home environment, noting the type of cars in the driveway, the noises in the other rooms, and any kitchen odors. Although an office at home provides convenience and tax benefits, it is a challenge for a beginner.

How to decorate your office is your call. For obvious reasons, it's preferable to avoid pictures with violent, sexual, or distressing themes. More neutral art is less distracting. My supervisors' offices are all unique. One is decorated in an English romantic design with intricate needlepoint, overstuffed chairs, and fresh flowers. Another has abstract modern art in neutral colors with a few enlarged photos of European landmarks. To minimize distraction, a third does not decorate the wall across from his patient's chair. Clearly, there is more than one way to create an office; and creating a space in which you feel comfortable is important.

THE FIRST FEW MOMENTS OF THE INITIAL SESSION

Sallie Gane settles into her chair and sneezes. She looks expectantly at me to start.

While later in therapy the patient will start talking about whatever is on her mind, it is my responsibility to start the first session if the patient does not know how to begin. My opening question will set the tone for the initial first meeting. While none of the beginnings that follow are "bad," some facilitate a discussion better than others.

EXAMPLE 2.2

Starting the session with a statement that may set the stage for a paternalistic relationship rather than a collaboration

THERAPIST: How can I help you?

SALLIE: I don't know actually. My friend told me I should be in therapy, but nothing is really wrong, I guess.

THERAPIST: Oh, why are you here then?

At first glance, the introductory question "How can I help you?" seems neutral and unassuming, but this opening may subtly promise quick relief of long-standing symptoms, a service that the therapist may not be able to provide. By suggesting a relationship based on dependence or paternalism—or maternalism—the question may set the stage for an undesirable regression if the patient expects a different type of process than the one that will actually occur.

Psychotherapy is not effective because the clinician administers a healing elixir to a passive patient. Instead, the power of the treatment lies in the collaboration between therapist and patient, with the patient acting as expert on the subject at hand, herself.

Unlike many other medical treatments, psychotherapy tends to be a slow process that doesn't follow a "Take two and call me in the morning" model. There is no potion that will rapidly alleviate emotional pain, provide a stable romantic relationship, or supply career motivation. Even most psychotropic medications, if indicated, do not work immediately. Understandably, most patients hope for a quick cure, but since this is usually not possible, a more neutral opening may be more appropriate.

Here's another opener that might lead to some trouble.

EXAMPLE 2.3

Starting the session with a statement that may make the patient defensive

THERAPIST: Can you tell me what is troubling you?

SALLIE: Well, I don't know. I feel okay. I'm not really that bad really. I've had a bit of trouble at school lately, but maybe it isn't even out of the ordinary.

When asked "What is troubling you?" or its equivalent ("Can you tell me what's wrong?"), a patient is likely to respond by minimizing her concerns. For patients sensitive to the stigma of mental health treatment, this innocuous question may have a humiliating sting. An opening question without an affective slant is preferable.

EXAMPLE 2.4

Starting the session with a statement that may facilitate discussion

THERAPIST: Can you tell me what brings you in?

SALLIE: My mother! She just keeps bugging me to get some professional help.

THERAPIST: That could be uncomfortable. What does she keep bugging you about?

Although many patients will respond favorably when asked "What brings you in?" some, like Sallie in Example 2.4, may use this query as an opportunity to externalize, for example, "I don't have a problem. I'm here because my mother wants me to be in treatment." For other patients, this opener may feel too threatening as it may suggest the therapist's need to get right down to business before even saying hello. In Example 2.4, I respond empathically to Sallie's statement, and follow her lead. If it is easier for Sallie to talk about her mother's concerns rather than her own, this is also where I will initially focus.

Here's a tried and true opener that should avoid defensiveness.

EXAMPLE 2.5

Starting the session with a statement that should avoid defensiveness

THERAPIST: How would you like to start?

SALLIE: Umm, you mean, why am I here?

THERAPIST: Sure. What would you like to tell me?

SALLIE: Well, I don't know. . . . I guess my life has been kind of a mess lately.

THERAPIST: (concerned look) How so?

SALLIE: Well, this guy broke up with me 6 months ago, and instead of feeling better, little by little, I just feel worse. I just can't stop thinking about him. I thought the relationship was going really well when he broke it off. I still don't know what happened.

THERAPISTT: The breakup was unexpected?

SALLIE: Completely! There was no warning at all.

Example 2.5's opener is the least directive of the outlined choices, but, for a novice, it may also feel the most awkward. Like other "moves" unique to psychotherapy, it is likely to feel more comfortable after a little practice. It can also be used as a backup if "What brings you in?" results in a defensive stance.

Congratulations! You are ready to meet your first patient and to start the consultation process. Balancing the four goals of the next three sessions—responding empathically, evaluating patient safety, obtaining basic background information, and creating an alliance with the patient—is the focus of the next three chapters.

> **Key words:** anonymity, confidentiality, distraction, intrusion, office arrangement, office furnishing, psychotherapy, privacy, safety, suicidality, therapeutic alliance, working alliance

3

Initiating an Alliance and Assessing Safety

The goals of the first session are to respond empathically to the patient's distress, to initiate a therapeutic alliance, to assess the patient's safety and to explain the consultative procedure. Relevant information gathering can be interwoven among these four processes.

THE PURPOSE AND PROCEDURE OF THE CONSULTATION

Sallie began the first session by telling me about her recent breakup with her boyfriend, Charlie. Then she paused for a moment. "I've never felt this bad before in my whole life. So what do you I think I should do? Tell me how to handle this."

I hate it when my patients ask me for advice. It's too tempting to take the bait and respond: "Well, Sallie, I think you should keep busy and be nice to yourself." It isn't a bad answer. It's certainly well meaning. It's just unlikely to help.

By the time a patient makes her way to your office, she has undoubtedly received loads of suggestions. She's in your office because they didn't work. Psychodynamic psychotherapy is different because the work attempts to help a person from the inside out rather than from the outside in. The process is understandably slow, so now when a new patient asks me for a quick solution, I take the opportunity to discuss the process of the next three or four sessions.

I use the first few sessions with a new patient to learn more about her primary concern, to gather some history, and to organize a preliminary treatment plan. Since I do not know what type of psychological treatment is appropriate for a new patient, I consider these early sessions as consultation visits, not the beginning of psychotherapy. I use the word "consultation" to describe these meetings, rather than "evaluation," because the former term sounds less judgmental and still implies that the interaction is time-limited.

EXAMPLE 3.1

Framing the first three visits

SALLIE: I've never felt this bad before ever in my life. So what do you I think I should do?

THERAPIST: I realize that you feel distressed, but at this point, I need to know much more before I can offer a responsible recommendation. For example, what have you already tried to help you feel better during this difficult time?

SALLIE: I don't know. I've tried a lot of things, but obviously they didn't work or I wouldn't be here in the first place! I assumed you would know how to make me feel better.

THERAPIST: Perhaps you feel disappointed that I need to understand you better before we can find a course of action that will help.

SALLIE: I am disappointed. I am sick of feeling so terrible. Well, whatever. What do you want to know?

THERAPIST: Feeling terrible for a long time is very upsetting. At this point, I think I can be most helpful to you if I hear more about your experience with Charlie and also learn a bit about your background.

SALLIE: Then what?

THERAPIST: I usually view these first few meetings as a consultation. It is an opportunity for me to learn more about you and to see if I can help, and for you to see whether you feel comfortable working with me. Together, by the end of the three or four visits, we should be able to come up with a preliminary treatment plan for this difficult situation. How does that sound to you?

SALLIE: Okay, I guess.

THERAPIST: Would it be okay if I jot down a few notes while you talk?

SALLIE: Sure. The last few months have been the worst of my life.

THERAPIST: If it isn't too painful, could you tell more about how they have been the worst in your life [*using Sallie's words to facilitate her associations*]?

SALLIE: Well, I haven't been sleeping or eating very well. I just feel mopey. I'm studying business at college; I'm a junior now. Usually I can focus really well, but for weeks now, my concentration has been shot.

Once the first few sessions are labeled as a consultation, they acquire a structure and a purpose. Patients may also be reassured when they learn that attendance at one therapy meeting does not commit them to a lengthy treatment course.

Although I don't take notes during an ongoing psychotherapy, I write down some basic facts, names, and dates (rather than record what the patient says verbatim) during the consultation. These pieces of information help me organize the patient's story into a a cohesive written summary. I will keep a copy for my records and, with permission, will forward a copy at the end of the consultation if I refer Sallie to another clinician.

The three- to four-visit consultation outlines an exit for both parties in case the therapist and patient are a poor match. (See Chapter 1 for a more detailed discussion of the patient–therapist match.) If the patient feels seriously uncomfortable with the clinician, she is encouraged to find another one, with the therapist's blessing. While it is the consultant's responsibility to provide treatment recommendations and referrals at the end of the consultation, she is not obligated to continue as a patient's therapist once the consultation is completed.

As I mentioned earlier, although most patients cooperate with the consultation format, many patients, like Sallie Gane, will request faster relief than psychotherapy can promise. Psychotherapy can't be rushed. In response to patients' impatience, I have learned innumerable ways to say "It is hard to tolerate delay and to keep working on this problem, but our ability to understand will help us come up with a reasonable course of action." (Please see Chapter 4 for another example.)

As a novice, I found it difficult to have confidence in my work and to convince my patients of therapy's efficacy when I hadn't personally experienced how psychotherapy could transform a person's life. Even with personal experience in one's own treatment, it may feel difficult to trust in one's own ability as a clinician to heal.

With time, as I saw my patients improve, it became easier to feel confident about my work. Skepticism was sometimes even advantageous when I used it to guide my learning in supervision. We hope our readers who are uncertain about the usefulness of psychotherapy can suspend disbelief as they give the treatment time to take effect. Clinical research and experience has shown that patients improve when therapy is practiced well. Just as patients need patience while they grapple with their problems in therapy, it is equally important that trainees are patient with themselves as they learn to practice this difficult but rewarding profession.

DIRECTING THE FIRST INTERVIEW

After mapping out the consultation process to a new patient, it is the therapist's responsibility to direct the first interview. After experimenting with many approaches in the last few years, I think the first meeting works best if my only goals are to establish a therapeutic alliance with the patient and to complete a suicide assessment, if that seems necessary. Experienced supervisors often say that a major point of a first session is to set the stage for a second session. If my patient doesn't feel understood and heard in the first meeting, she might never return.

It is easy enough to state how important it is to establish a therapeutic alliance during the beginning of a psychotherapy, but as a novice I bristled at this sort of statement because it seemed too vague and theoretical. To avoid making this mistake, we will outline some specific strategies later in this chapter that you can use to create a therapeutic alliance. First, we'll offer some examples of how the process can go awry.

To foster a therapeutic alliance, the therapist needs to be responsive but not overbearing, although this is always easier said than done. As a beginner, it is easy to under- or overdirect the first session. We'll offer an example of each.

EXAMPLE 3.2

The therapist takes an overly passive stance during the first interview

SALLIE: Well, I haven't been sleeping or eating very well. . . . My concentration has been shot.

THERAPIST: So you haven't been eating very well?

SALLIE: Yeah. I'm not hungry at all. I have to force myself to eat, but all food tastes like sawdust to me. Half the time I just feel sick to my stomach. The only thing that tastes good to me is ice cream.

THERAPIST: Hmm. . . .

SALLIE: Last night, I spent the evening watching TV for 3 hours, and eating a pint of chocolate chip cookie dough ice cream for dinner. Gross, isn't it? I just feel like crap most of the day.

THERAPIST: Yes. . . .

SALLIE: Last week, I sat at home and cried all day long. That's been happening every now and then. I realized that I had to do something, so I made this appointment.

Example 3.2 illustrates a very traditional psychoanalytic approach to the first session. I avoid directing the interview in any way as I listen to Sallie's associations. Years ago, many first sessions were conducted with this approach. While the psychotherapist may have asked a few questions of the patient, in general, she would intrude as little as possible. The patient would associate freely, saying whatever came to mind. According to theory, the less the therapist hindered the patient's train of thought, the more likely the patient would reach important repressed material.

From this traditional perspective, questions by the psychoanalytic psychotherapist were not seen as useful, but as unwanted influences that would taint the psychotherapeutic process. The goal for the therapist was to be as neutral as possible, and the metaphor of therapist as a blank slate was introduced. As a result, in worst instances, a therapist could treat a patient for years and not know if she had experienced self-injurious impulses, had a serious head injury, had recovered from leukemia as a child, and so on, unless the patient chose to volunteer this information.

Spontaneous association continues to be a powerful source of information that therapists should employ, especially after the consultation is completed and the psychodynamic psychotherapy begins (please see Chapters 6 and 14), but we do not recommend a pervasively nondirective approach during diagnostic sessions. Moreover, the free association strategy is also not as neutral as it may have once seemed. It is impossible to attain a true "blank slate" status. In fact, a therapist who does not ask questions or respond to her patient in a human way is often perceived as odd or withholding rather than as neutrally listening.

In an attempt to avoid the "blank slate" approach, a beginner might overorganize the first session around a list of predetermined questions. It is understandably easy to overshoot and to become more directive than necessary with this strategy.

EXAMPLE 3.3

An overstructured approach for the first interview

SALLIE: Well, I haven't been sleeping or eating very well. . . . My concentration has been shot.

THERAPIST: So, your eating, sleeping, and concentration have all been affected? Is it sometimes hard to motivate as well?

SALLIE: Yes.

THERAPIST: It sounds as though this has been be a difficult time. Have you been feeling hopeless at all?

SALLIE: Sometimes.

THERAPIST: Hmm (*sympathetically*). Some people who feel hopeless start thinking a lot about dying or wishing that they were dead? Has this been part of your experience?

SALLIE: Oh, no. I'm Catholic. I could never do anything to hurt myself.

THERAPIST: So you haven't thought of hurting yourself at all?

SALLIE: Nah.

THERAPIST: Have you ever felt this bad before?

In Example 3.3, the approach to the first psychotherapeutic interview is modeled after a first visit with an internist or family physician. Symptoms are identified, their severity is clarified, and data are gathered with the intent of making a diagnosis. Many of the questions require only short, one-word answers. The therapist is able to make a possible diagnosis of a major depression by identifying five neurovegetative symptoms in less than 5 minutes.

While this approach has a number of disadvantages for relatively stable patients, for some individuals this interview style is the structure of choice. If the patient lacks some internal structure due to psychosis, mania, substance abuse, or comparable conditions, a structured interview will compensate for the deficiency. The increased organization will provide comfort for the out-of-control patient. By acting as a diagnostician, the therapist can effectively begin to clarify the problem and to plan an emergency treatment strategy. In a sense, this interview follows the format of an emergency room psychiatric interview or a psychopharmacological consultation. (For more information on how to respond to a psychiatric emergency, see Chapter 9.)

A more structured interviewing style may also come in handy if your new patient becomes tongue-tied during the first interview. With an empathic statement such as "Perhaps you find it hard to think of what to say because it's such a troubling and complicated topic. Let's take a breather and I'll fill in some other information I need," you can use the first session to gather as much history as you would like.

We have included a sample questionnaire at the end of Chapter 4 that summarizes the information you'll need by the end of the consultation. I have used the questionnaire in two ways. If my patient is at a loss for words during the consultation, I may use the questionnaire to guide my interview. I've also given a patient a copy of the questionnaire at the end of the first session to fill out and to return to me at or before the second session.

It is important to know how to employ a structured interview for disorganized patients or for those who feel uncomfortable talking spontaneously during the first session, but for most new patients an intensive history taking during the first session can hinder the development of a therapeutic alliance. For the majority of people entering your office for the first time, an interested approach that balances an ability to listen, a capacity to follow the patient's associations, and the foresight to assess suicidality is most likely to preserve safety while also fostering a therapeutic alliance

EXAMPLE 3.4

Balancing the need for information and the need to create a therapeutic alliance during the first consultation session

SALLIE: Well, I haven't been sleeping or eating very well. . . . My concentration has been shot.

THERAPIST: Can you tell me more about what has been going on?

SALLIE: Well, I usually am so full of energy. Now I just don't care. This Saturday, for instance, I just stayed in my room and listened to music. I'm such a loser lately. I mean, the weather has been so perfect, and I'm listening to love songs crying my eyes out. What a mess!

THERAPIST: A lot of sadness and distress. Do you have an understanding of what has made it so hard?

SALLIE: For starters, I still can't believe that Charlie broke up with me. BOOM! It seemed out of nowhere. I didn't anticipate it at all, and he didn't really give me a reason. Well, he did talk about one thing that bothered him. . . .

THERAPIST: What was that?

SALLIE: I don't know—maybe something about my tone of voice. Sometimes, he would complain that I was bossing him around when I was just telling him my opinion. It just doesn't make any sense to me. I'm a very sensitive person, and with Charlie I was always on my best behavior. And it's the first time I've ever really liked a guy this much. Usually, I am the one to break it off. (*Reaches for a tissue.*)

THERAPIST: When did this happen?

SALLIE: About 6 months ago.

THERAPIST: Six months of grief: I can see that Charlie really meant a lot to you. Can you tell me more about the relationship and breakup?

SALLIE: I thought he was "it." He seemed perfect from the first moment I laid eyes on him. Our first 2 weeks together were perfect. He was perfect—cute, smart, funny, nice. After the first few weeks though, it was never the same. He is majoring in music, and there really isn't any future in that, so I tried to convince him to change to an economics major, like me. He seemed interested at first, but then he started to withdraw and not answer my phone calls. I don't understand it, because I was just trying to help him out, and he knew it. I don't know if that was the beginning of the end. I have no idea why he was so sensitive about my suggestions. We were together a couple of months, and then he said he wasn't interested anymore. It was so cruel, because just weeks before he said he was in love with me. I don't know what I did wrong, but obviously, I'm a total failure.

THERAPIST: That sounds harsh. It is very painful when a relationship that seems so promising doesn't work out. Somehow it feels to you that you are a failure because of the breakup? What do you mean?

SALLIE: If I were really capable, I could have made this work. And it feels so strange to be the one who was rejected. See, like I said, I am the person who ends relationships. I've had two serious relationships before Charlie. They were nice guys, but maybe too nice. I don't know, they just seemed so young. They did whatever I wanted them to do, then I'd get bored and break it off. Charlie was different; he was independent. He had his own ideas, and somehow I messed it up, and I don't know how. I was just trying to help him when I gave him career advice. I feel like I can't do anything right. How did I manage to ruin such a good thing?

THERAPIST: It feels to you that it is all your fault?

SALLIE: Yes, completely. Sometimes I just want to curl up and sleep all day just to avoid the pain.

THERAPIST: It does sound as though you have been in a lot of pain. Sometimes when a person feels so hopeless, she might think about dying or wishing she were dead. Has that been a part of your experience?

SALLIE: Oh, I'm Catholic. I could never do anything to hurt myself.

THERAPIST: Had it crossed your mind?

SALLIE: A couple of times. Well, not exactly. I don't care if my plane fly-
ing home from vacation drops from the sky or if I don't wake up in
the morning, but I would never purposely hurt myself.

In Example 3.4, I use a balanced approach: following Sallie's narra-
tive, empathizing with her situation, and inserting a suicide assessment
in response to Sallie's hopelessness. Example 3.4 follows the patient's
lead, in contrast to Example 3.3, which leads the patient. The question
regarding suicide fits easily within the context of the conversation,
rather than within a predetemined review of the neurovegetive signs
and symptoms of depression. With the approach used in Example 3.4, I
may not complete the full psychiatric review of systems within the first
session, but by helping Sallie describe her experience, I can empathize
with her most urgent concerns.

HELPFUL HINTS: HOW TO LISTEN AND HOW
TO CULTIVATE A THERAPEUTIC ALLIANCE

Over time, I've learned a few specific techniques that help cultivate a
therapeutic alliance. First, I ask detailed questions about the patient's
main concern. If the patient tells me a few facts and then stops short
(i.e., "I am upset about my breakup with my boyfriend"), I flesh out the
story with questions like "Could you tell me more?" or statements such
as "Please go on."

Second, I ask every patient why she decided to come into treatment
at this particular time. In Sallie's case, she has been suffering for 6
months. What led her to come in today, rather than last week or next
week? I am almost guaranteed to learn more about a patient's present
conflicts and concerns with this inquiry.

Third, if it doesn't feel right to follow a patient's emotional statement with a question, I respond with a validating comment that
reframes what the patient is sharing without diminishing its intensity.
For example, when Sallie says, "I don't known what I did wrong. . . .
I'm a total failure!" I tune into her emotional state by naming it: "That
sounds harsh. It is very painful when a relationship that seems so promising doesn't work out. Somehow it feels to you that you are a failure because of the breakup? What do you mean?"

The ability to listen empathically is one of the most powerful tools
of an effective therapist. Even so, I spent my training years missing
empathic opportunities and fighting against an internal pull toward
"fix-it" statements. Again and again I'd hear paragraphs flow out of my
mouth full of well-intentioned advice and cheerful pick-me-ups: "It

wasn't your fault that it didn't work out. Charlie didn't sound that nice anyway. I'm sure there are plenty more guys out there whom you could date."

I would have been the master if fix-it statements were helpful. They aren't. Minimizing emotional pain and distracting people from their discomfort may actually exacerbate emotional distress. As a therapist, I am most useful if I tune into my patient's unique experience and don't assume I know how to fix her crisis. I now think of empathic listening that avoids minimization as a genuine way to "fix it." With this tool, my patient will feel understood, and emotional pain may slowly abate.

The therapeutic alliance is also nurtured by reminding the patient that she and the therapist are working together toward a common goal: the patient's health, recovery, or resolution of problems. This is accomplished by using first person plural pronouns such as "we," "us," or "our" when referring to the work, task, process, or goal of therapy. (Example: Our work together is to find out what would be the best course of action for you.)

This strategy is further reinforced by explaining my questions to the patient. For example: "I'm asking these questions about your family history because it helps me put your current difficulties in context, and because a vulnerability to depression may continue from generation to generation."

With these five tools in my back pocket—asking questions about the material important to the patient; inquiring "why now?"; validating affect; framing the consultation as "our task"; and explaining the consultation procedure as it unfolds—I can cultivate a therapeutic alliance within the first few sessions. Framing the therapy.

ASSESSING SUICIDALITY

Whatever style you choose to employ during the consultation, you must complete a suicide assessment during the first interview if your patient seems to be at any risk for self-harm. In Sallie's case, I screen early for suicidality because she has many symptoms of depression. Other risk factors for self-harm include substance abuse, psychosis, bereavement, HIV positive status or other illness, loss of employment, borderline personality disorder, mania, panic disorder with agoraphobia, perceived abandonment, or divorce.

If a new patient doesn't have any risk factors for self-harm and she has a clear focus on her future, asking about suicidality may be in response to the clinician's needs rather than the patient's. However, if I am at all unsure about the patient's self-destuctive impulses, I will ask.

Many suicidal patients will discuss their self-destructive impulses honestly when asked directly, but few will spontaneously offer this information. (For more detail on how to complete a suicide assessment for a patient who is currently at risk, please see Chapter 9.)

A suicide assessment is the only part of the psychiatric consultation that should not be postponed to future meetings if the patient has any risk factors. A large proportion of successful suicides are preceded by contacts with the health system. Quiet calls for help are often not heard. In addition, the diagnosis of depression, a major antecedent to suicide, is frequently overlooked by many medical professionals who aren't schooled in mental health. Despite all these reasons supporting the inclusion of a suicide assessment in the first meeting, it is easy for therapists to "forget" to complete this portion of the evaluation, because it is understandably discomforting to ask about this topic. However, ignoring it may prove fatal.

COLLECTING BASIC INFORMATION
AT THE END OF THE FIRST SESSION

About 20 minutes before my first consultation session with Sallie draws to a close, I collect some administrative information and then shift the subject back to Sallie's main concern 10 minutes before the hour ends.

EXAMPLE 3.5

Collecting some basic information at the end of the first session

THERAPIST: The situation with Charlie has clearly been a tough one. We will definitely talk about it more, but I need to take time now to collect some information for my records.

SALLIE: Okay. What do you need to know?

THERAPIST: Well, for starters, what is your address? [*I need to collect this information in the first session if it was not gathered during the previous phone contacts.*]

SALLIE: I live at 1111 Central Street in Boston.

THERAPIST: What is the zip code?

SALLIE: Oh, it is 02114.

THERAPIST: If I ever needed to call you about scheduling changes, should I call the number you left on my machine last week?

SALLIE: Yeah. You can reach me easily there. I also do some work-study at the library. I can give you that number as well if you'd like.

THERAPIST: If I call the home number, would it be better if I don't identify myself as a doctor?

SALLIE: Actually, that's a good point. It's my private line, but sometimes I listen to new messages with people around. If you don't mind, it would be easier if you didn't identify yourself as a doctor. Is that okay?

THERAPIST: Many people feel that way, which is why I ask. I also like to have the phone number of someone to contact in case of an emergency.

SALLIE: What do you mean?

THERAPIST: Well, overall, I take the confidentiality of my patients very seriously. If anyone ever called me and asked if you were seeing me, I wouldn't divulge this information without your written permission. But in case you are ever at very high risk of hurting yourself or someone else, I would like to have an emergency contact.

SALLIE: Oh, I don't think you'll ever need to call anyone, but I guess I should give you my parents' number. Their names are Jane and Anthony Gane. They live in Framingham.

THERAPIST: I don't expect emergencies either, but I want you to know the procedures I follow if one should arise. Also, I want to tell you about my training and my supervision.

As you know, this is a teaching hospital, and I'll be in training here for the next 2 years. One of the advantages of receiving your care here is that trainees like me receive advice regularly from experienced, fully trained clinicians. To obtain that guidance, I'll have to give my supervisor information about you.

It's not unusual to have some questions about this process. How does it sound to you?

SALLIE: I don't know. I don't really want anyone else to know what we talk about.

THERAPIST: Can you tell me what you are concerned about?

SALLIE: What will they think of me? I don't want anyone to know my business.

THERAPIST: I understand your wish for privacy. It's important that you know that my supervisors are required by law to keep the information that I share with them confidential.

Their presence will benefit both of us. With their help, I will be able to provide you with the most comprehensive treatment.

SALLIE: They don't tell anyone else?

THERAPIST: That's right. The discussions I have with my supervisor are private.

SALLIE: I don't know. I've never really heard of anything like this, but I guess it makes sense if I think about it. Whatever. I don't love it, but I guess it's okay.

THERAPIST: If you have any further questions about it, please don't hesitate to ask me.

Let's see, I also want to let you know how to get in touch with me if you need to contact me between sessions. I have a voicemail answering system and a beeper. I check my messages many times a day on weekdays and about once a day on weekends. During the week, I'll always try to answer a message within 24 hours. If you need to contact me in an emergency, my pager is on 24 hours a day. I can't always answer right away, and there may even be a delay of an hour or two, but I'll answer as soon as I can. If the emergency can't wait that long, please don't wait for my return call but go to the nearest emergency room for treatment.

SALLIE: Oh, okay. But, like I said, I don't expect any real emergencies.

THERAPIST: Let's see if we can find a time to meet these next few weeks. Are you free Wednesdays at 4:00?

SALLIE: Let me look at my schedule book. Yeah, I think I can do that.

THERAPIST: You may already know this, but therapy differs from other medical visits because you can depend on it to start and end on time. Each session will last 50 minutes.

SALLIE: (*Nods.*) Okay.

THERAPIST: Okay. I think that is all the administrative information I need to cover. We need to stop in a few minutes, but I was wondering how has this meeting felt to you? What has it felt like to talk about these concerns with me?

SALLIE: I don't know really. It feels weird. I am more a listener than a talker usually, and 50 minutes can seem a bit long.

THERAPIST: Do you feel uncomfortable?

SALLIE: A little.

THERAPIST: Enough to keep you from coming back?

SALLIE: I don't think so. I really need help with this, and it hasn't been getting better on its own.

THERAPIST: I am glad you could share this with me. Consultation sessions are different from a discussion with a concerned friend or relative because our goal is to focus completely on your concerns. It can feel different at first. You may have more feelings about this session before our next one, and I would be interested in hearing what your thoughts are next time.

SALLIE: Okay.

THERAPIST: Before you leave, I want to give you a questionnaire to help gather information rapidly. You can fill it out and mail it to me or bring it to our next appointment. How does that sound to you?

SALLIE: That's fine.

THERAPIST: I know that you're more concerned about what happened with Charlie than you are about any of these background matters. Let's use the remaining time to talk about him.

In this chapter, we present Sallie as a clinic patient to demonstrate how to talk about supervision with a patient. As the clinic handles the finances, I do not need to discuss fees and payment. In Chapter 8, Sallie is a private patient and we illustrate how to negotiate a fee and discuss insurance as part of the first session.

As shown in Example 3.5, I use this session to educate Sallie about the 50-minute session. Some therapists work in 45-minute blocks, which is an acceptable alternative. I've found it's easiest to specify the session's length early in the process. Without this discussion, Sallie may not understand why I stop the session 10 minutes before the hour.

Near the end the session, I also check how Sallie has experienced the meeting. Sometimes a new patient will use this opportunity to share her ambivalence about therapy, as Sallie did. Interestingly enough, once a patient has voiced her uncertainty, she may actually be more likely to return for the second session. I praise Sallie's ability to talk openly about our interaction to encourage future discourse on the topic. She is likely to experience more feelings about our meeting, and now she might feel comfortable sharing them with me.

In summary, I try to accomplish four major tasks for a successful first session. If I hear the patient's distress empathically, explain the consultation process, assess suicidality if necessary, and concentrate on forming an alliance with the patient, the consultation is well on its way.

Key words: abandonment, data gathering, diagnosis, empathy, interview, loss, psychiatric emergencies, psychotherapy evaluation, rapport, rejection, risk assessment, safety, suicide, therapeutic alliance

4

Enhancing the Therapeutic Alliance and Eliciting History

By asking the patient how she is experiencing the process of the consultation, and by explaining the relevance of psychiatric and medical history, the clinician reinforces the therapeutic alliance. The second session is also the therapist's opportunity to collect some basic psychiatric and medical information. Time must be reserved at the end of the session to talk about the patient's primary concern.

THE BEGINNING OF THE SECOND SESSION

When Sallie returns for her second session, I start to feel a little more confident. With the knowledge that our therapeutic alliance is off to a good start, it's easier for me to be more directive during our second session. I'll use the time to outline Sallie's medical and psychiatric history, but before I start the data collection, I ask Sallie about her week and her experience of our first meeting.

EXAMPLE 4.1

Opening the second session

Sallie walks briskly into the room and sits down. She looks at me expectantly.

SALLIE: How are you, Dr. Bender?

THERAPIST: I'm all right, thanks. How are you doing?

SALLIE: Okay, I guess.

THERAPIST: Any thoughts about our last meeting? How did it feel to you?

SALLIE: It was fine, I guess. Well, to be honest, I don't love the idea of coming in to talk to a stranger about my personal problems, but I can't stand to feel this way anymore, so I'm willing to try anything. I did hear from Charlie this week—that was a highlight (*sarcastically*). He needed a book that he'd left at my dorm. We talked for about 30 seconds. Nothing about missing me or about wondering if breaking up was the right decision. He's doing fine, and I'm so messed up that I need to see a shrink to get over him.

THERAPIST: It's clear that the breakup with Charlie has been a very painful experience. Can you tell me more about how you feel "messed up?"

SALLIE: I don't know. At the beginning of last week, I actually felt a little better. Maybe talking to you did help a tiny bit. But then, after his call, I was back to square one. I didn't sleep that night, and my stomach was in knots all week. I've always looked down on women who get all riled up about a relationship, and now look at me. I'm so pathetic.

THERAPIST: Aren't you overly harsh with yourself?

SALLIE: I don't think so. I am pathetic.

THERAPIST: When you start feeling upset about Charlie, how do you take the edge off the pain?

SALLIE: I call my friend Gwen a lot. She's been helpful, mainly because she keeps me busy. It helps a little bit, I guess. But, Dr. Bender (*in a slightly irritated tone*), I've been trying to feel better for weeks, doing a million different activities, and nothing really works. I've taken aerobics, gone running, biking, hiking . . . you name it. Like I said, I'm here because I don't feel better, no matter what I do.

THERAPIST: (*naming the emotion that Sallie is expressing*) Has it been a frustrating experience—trying so hard to feel better but then continuing to feel so upset?

SALLIE: (*Relaxes into her seat.*) EXACTLY!

THERAPIST: I think it's a wise idea to consider therapy at this time to understand more about the situation with Charlie and to understand why it has been so hard to move on. In the next couple of sessions, I'll need to get to know you better in order to come up with a treatment plan that feels reasonable to both of us. I'd like to use part of this meeting to learn about your medical and psychiatric history.

SALLIE: (*aggravated*) With all due respect, Dr. Bender, I need to get better as fast as possible. Do we have to spend time talking about stuff that isn't bothering me right now?

THERAPIST: It makes sense that you want to get better as quickly as possible. I need to know your medical history because some medical conditions intensify emotional distress and interfere with recovery.

SALLIE: (*Interrupts.*) Well, I'm not here to be analyzed. I just need to get over this stupid guy. I don't think it will be that helpful to talk about my past and my first memory and all those Freudian things I learned about in my freshman psych class.

THERAPIST: I'm sorry to be adding to your frustration, but in order to come up with a useful treatment plan, I need to know a bit more about you. To begin to understand your pain with Charlie, I need to know more about you as an individual.

SALLIE: Okay, whatever (*sighs*), how long do you think this will take?

THERAPIST: Let's see how it goes, but the consultation usually takes three or four sessions.

SALLIE: Well, what do you want to know?

THERAPIST: Well, for starters, I want to clarify how this breakup has affected your ability to function in school. Have you been able to keep up with your classwork despite feeling so poorly?

Before I focus on information collection during the second session, I model and encourage direct and honest communication by asking Sallie how she experienced our first meeting. The wording of my questions ("Any *thoughts* about our last meeting? How did it *feel* to you?") purposely pulls for both cognition and affect. In general, it is less challenging to share one's thoughts than one's underlying emotions. As treatment progresses, the focus on affect will become more intense, but early in the consultation, my line of questioning offers Sallie a choice.

As Sallie starts to relate the events of her week, I strategically ask specific details of her experience. Sometimes the questions themselves use words from Sallie's previous statements. For instance, when Sallie mentions that she feels so "messed up," I respond, "Can you tell me more about how you feel 'messed up'?"

Sallie becomes irritated when I focus, even for a moment, on her coping mechanisms rather than her distress. Her response is a cue to change tactics. When I validate how helpless she has felt, she visibly relaxes and becomes more agreeable.

Fortunately, most patients aren't as ornery as Sallie so the second interview is rarely this emotionally taxing. But, as a novice, I was most worried about patients who would question my judgment and leave me tongue-tied. Surprisingly, while Dr. Messner and I wrote this book and I grappled with Sallie's feisty nature, my confidence increased. Now, because of my experience with my virtual patient, I feel more competent dealing with the flesh and blood variety. Basically, if you are ready for a "Salliesque" patient, many other patients will feel easy by comparison.

A MORE DIRECTIVE APPROACH

In order to gather the necessary medical and psychiatric information for a comprehensive consultation, I am more directive during the second session. Nowadays I don't have trouble switching gears (following the patient's lead in Session 1 and leading the patient in Session 2), but this change in approach was not easy for me to master. Early on, I worried that I was squelching the patient's self-expression every time I directed the questioning away from the present complaint and toward pertinent history. In my attempt to be the ultimate empathic therapist, I often completed the consultation without obtaining essential historical data.

My inability to redirect also led to a few embarrassing moments in supervision when I didn't know fundamental facts about patients I had seen for months. Supervisors would encourage me to acquire this information as soon as possible, but if I was bad at interrupting a new patient during the first few visits, I was even worse at interrupting a patient in ongoing therapy. It took time to experience the treatment benefit of a comprehensive consultation, and only then did I feel empowered to direct the interview during the first few sessions.

To formulate the most informed treatment plan, a clinician needs to obtain a medical and psychiatric history from every new patient *whether or not the therapist has medical training*. Unrecognized physical disease may first present as psychological distress, and physical illness can have a profound emotional effect on a patient's life.

For medical questions about the patient's current symptoms, I refer the patient to an internist. Dr. Messner once treated a 45-year-old lawyer, whom we will call Mr. Harper, who started psychotherapy because of generalized anxiety with intermittent panic attacks following an unexpected promotion. As psychotherapists, it's easy to formulate a whole bunch of different hypotheses as to why success might feel overwhelming to a man in his 40s, but during the consultation interview, Dr. Messner also learned that the patient had a family history of heart disease. The patient's father had died of a heart attack at 46. While this fact may have psychodynamic importance in the treatment of a 45-year-old man, the medical implications are more urgent. Had Mr. Harper seen his internist in the last year? No. Did his panic attacks include symptoms of chest pain and shortness of breath? Yes. A possibly life-saving intervention at the beginning of psychiatric treatment was a referral to an internist for a physical exam and cardiac workup. Happily, Mr. Harper's cardiac condition was deemed non-life-threatening. However, especially in light of his family history, it was reassuring that a cardiologist would continue to follow him as needed. If Dr. Messner had taken a "free-floating" approach to the consultation sessions, the necessary medical intervention would not have occurred. While physicians will be understandably more comfortable talking to their patients about health issues, nonphysicians can be very effective if they refer psychotherapy patients for a medical consultation whenever a patient is suffering from a bothersome physical symptom that hasn't been evaluated by a medical doctor.

Our consultation questionnaire at the end of this chapter screens for medical symptoms that may require follow-up. For positive answers noted in the "Brief Review of Symptoms" section, the therapist should refer the patient to her primary care physician for further investigation.

STRATEGY FOR THE SECOND SESSION

During the second session, I focus on the details of the psychiatric and medical history and only ask about other historical information if extra time is available. I use the consultation questionnaire at the end of this chapter to guide my interview by using it as a cribsheet during the sessions or by asking my patient to fill it out between sessions. (You have permission to reproduce this form.)

Every now and then, a new patient feels that her current concerns are so urgent that she is unable to focus exclusively on her history during the second session. When this occurs, I quickly scan the completed questionnaire during our meeting, and then review the answers in more detail during the third and fourth session. Or, if I plan to continue to work with the patient after the consultation, I may use 15–20 minutes of several sessions to collect the necessary historical information.

EXAMPLE 4.2

Clarifying the patient's current psychiatric symptoms—a more directive approach in the second consultation session

THERAPIST: Well, for starters, I wanted to clarify how this breakup has affected your ability to function in school. Have you been able to keep up with your classwork despite feeling so poorly?

SALLIE: Well, even though I have felt crappy most of the time, I haven't fallen behind in my classes. School is the only thing I am successful at nowadays.

THERAPIST: It is impressive that despite your distress you have been able to continue your work. Have you been able to spend time with friends as well? You mentioned a friend, Gwen. . . .

SALLIE: Yes, Gwen has been great. She calls me every day to check on me, and we go see a lot of movies together. It gets my mind off things.

THERAPIST: She has been a help to you?

SALLIE: Yes.

THERAPIST: Has anyone else been helpful during this difficult time?

SALLIE: My family, I guess. They are supportive of me, but I don't usually tell them details about my love life, you know.

THERAPIST: I want to get a good sense of how the breakup has affected your life in many areas. Last week we talked briefly about your sleep and appetite, but I wanted to touch base on this again. How well have you slept the last few weeks?

SALLIE: It's erratic. Sometimes I have a lot of trouble getting to bed, but I would say that most nights I probably get about 8 hours of sleep.

THERAPIST: And your appetite?

SALLIE: It's bad. I just don't feel like eating most of the time.

THERAPIST: Have you lost any weight?

SALLIE: No, I haven't actually. Too bad . . . it would be a little bonus. You know, get dumped and get skinny. (*Grins.*)

THERAPIST: [*I note that Sallie is apparently normal in weight for her height. My next questions screen for an eating disorder.*] Do you have any worries about eating?

SALLIE: Maybe a little. I'd like to be one size smaller at least.

THERAPIST: Have you ever put yourself on a very strict diet and tried to lose a lot of weight, although everyone else thought you looked okay?

SALLIE: Nah. I've never been that disciplined. I had a friend in high school who got obsessed with her weight and became way too skinny, but I could never do that. I'd get too hungry.

THERAPIST: Some students your age will eat a lot of food when they are very upset, but then they'll regret it afterwards and make themselves vomit. Sometimes they use a dangerous medication called ipecac. Have you ever struggled with bingeing or purging?

SALLIE: No, I never did that, but I don't really like to talk to people about this stuff.

THERAPIST: (*wondering if there is more to learn because of Sallie's reluctance to talk about this particular topic*) You'd be surprised how many people have trouble with food.

SALLIE: Well, I did take laxatives for about a week in high school because I felt really bloated.

THERAPIST: What else was going on then?

SALLIE: Nothing really important. I was applying to college and stressed about that, but mainly I felt fat and wanted to fit into this slinky dress for the prom.

THERAPIST: Sometimes people find it hard to stop taking laxatives once they start. How was it for you?

SALLIE: I don't think it was that big a deal. I did it for a little while— maybe a few weeks—but then I stopped.

THERAPIST: How did you manage to stop?

SALLIE: I don't know. I got weak, and then I stopped, okay? (*defensively*)

THERAPIST: I imagine it may have been a difficult time for you if you were using laxatives. All medications for weight loss can be addicting, so it takes a lot of internal motivation to be able to stop.

SALLIE: (*slightly calmer*) Yeah, it did.

THERAPIST: Because these products can affect a person's health, I do need to know about them. Have you ever used diet pills or diuretics to lose weight?

SALLIE: What are diuretics?

THERAPIST: Good question. They are medications that make a person urinate a lot and are used to treat high blood pressure, but sometimes people use them secretly to try to lose weight.

SALLIE: No, I never did that. I thought about taking diet pills, but I never did.

THERAPIST: What protected you?

SALLIE: I don't know. I am sensitive to caffeine. I knew these medications were related to speed, and I didn't want to feel all wound up. So, I avoided them.

THERAPIST: I ask these questions because a lot of women your age have some difficulty with eating. It sounds like you have struggled with this some in the past. How about now?

SALLIE: I'm better now, I think. Even though I have felt sort of sick to my stomach lately because I've been so upset, I'm not doing anything unhealthy to lose weight.

THERAPIST: Has your energy been affected as well?

SALLIE: Oh, I don't have much energy, especially when I don't eat much that day.

THERAPIST: These last few months certainly sound tough. Have you ever felt this bad before?

SALLIE: No, this is the worst I have ever felt.

THERAPIST: Overall, there are some symptoms that are making it difficult to function day to day, but somehow you have managed to keep up with school and friends?

SALLIE: Yes, I guess that is right.

THERAPIST: Can you correct me? What part doesn't feel right?

SALLIE: Well, even though I can still be sociable and still do well in school, I'm not doing well at all.

THERAPIST: Tell me if this is right. Even though you have been able to maintain your schoolwork and friendships, you still don't feel at all like yourself.

SALLIE: Yeah, that fits.

When a new patient reports significant dysphoria, I determine early on whether her current symptoms are consistent with a diagnosis of major depressive disorder, as outlined in DSM-IV. A useful mnemonic can organize your review: SIGECAPS. (This abbreviation could either stand for the name Sigmund E Caps or the abbreviated prescription for E capsules. It was devised by Cary Gross, MD.) Each letter stands for a neurovegetative symptom of depression: S, a change in *s*leep; I, a decrease in *i*nterest and pleasure; G, an increase in *g*uilt and hopelessness; E, a decrease in *e*nergy; C, a decrease in *c*oncentration; A, a change in *a*ppetite; P, *p*sychomotor retardation or agitation; and S, *s*uicidal thoughts, intentions, plans or actions. A person has major depressive disorder if she experiences five of the preceding symptoms for longer than 2 weeks in addition to a sad or irritable mood. Sallie has some symptoms of depression, although her interest, concentration, and sleep are basically intact.

For Sallie, a trial of psychotherapy without medications is reasonable, but if her symptoms worsen with treatment, a medication evaluation might be indicated. In general, if my new patient has any psychiatric symptom that significantly affects her daily functioning, I include a psychopharmacological evaluation as part of her consultation. Although it is beyond the scope of this book to review how to complete a psychopharmacological evaluation, we have listed a number of good references in the bibliography.

In Example 4.2, I also fold a number of questions about eating disorders into my SIGECAPS review. Eating disorders are especially prevalent in young women, but patients rarely offer information about food restriction or bulimia spontaneously. These disorders also deserve some special attention because they place a patient at medical risk. Among many other complications, anorexia nervosa can lead to osteoporosis and bone fractures, and bulimia nervosa can lead to cardiac dysrhythmias. Both conditions have significant mortality rates when they are untreated. If a patient is restricting food intake and appears significantly below a normal body weight or is actively bingeing or purging, she is best served by a treatment team that includes a therapist, internist, and nutritionist. For my complicated eating-disordered patients, I also intermittently review their treatment with an expert experienced in this specialty.

Ultimately, there is no way to be ready for every clinical situation. Over time, I've come to the conclusion that, even as a seasoned clinician, I will never know everything. No practioner does. However, if I recognize what I don't know and when I need consultation, I will be able to provide excellent, ethical care.

As I continue to ask questions about Sallie's psychiatric history, I might fall for Sallie's nonchalant and somewhat defensive attitude and make some erroneous nonempathic assumptions about her past.

EXAMPLE 4.3

The therapist assumes incorrect information about the patient

THERAPIST: So, let me review some past psychiatric history. You probably haven't seen a psychiatrist before, have you?

SALLIE: Actually, I have.

THERAPIST: As a child?

SALLIE: No, actually it was just a few years ago, but I didn't want to go.

When faced with a question that assumes a particular response— such as "You probably haven't seen a psychiatrist before, have you?"—a self-conscious patient may minimize or edit her history in order to present a good impression. For the patient to feel safe sharing private and potentially shaming information, the clinician needs to create a non-judgmental atmosphere and avoid "leading the witness."

Clinical experience with a wide range of patients has helped me avoid erroneous clinical assumptions. When I started residency, I minimized the psychopathology in college students like Sallie Gane. After a few years, my assessments became more accurate, but I proceeded to make the same mistakes all over again in my private practice. If the patient was the least bit intimidating (a lawyer, another mental health professional, a wealthy and/or attractive patient), I was at risk for "leading the witness," as I did in Example 4.3. Again, clinical experience decreased my anxiety, and my clinical acumen improved.

Here's Take 2 with an approach that helps Sallie share her experience.

EXAMPLE 4.4

Collecting a personal and family psychiatric history

THERAPIST: So, have you ever seen a therapist before?

SALLIE: Well, when I was in high school, I saw someone for about a year.

THERAPIST: How did you experience the treatment?

SALLIE: Actually, even though I didn't want to go at first, I ended up liking Dr. Anders. He was a nice guy, and I always felt better after talking to him. It was a good experience.

THERAPIST: Can you tell me why you started seeing Dr. Anders?

SALLIE: Well, actually, it was around the time that I was using the laxatives.

THERAPIST: What was going on?

SALLIE: Well, I was really stressed out. I was trying to decide which college to go to, and my parents were totally invested in my attending the state university. I don't know. I just got overwhelmed with the whole idea, so I started to focus on the prom to keep my mind off of graduation, and moving on. You know, the whole growing-up thing. Dr. Anders helped me figure this out.

I had this great black dress to wear to the prom, but it was a little too tight when I bought it. Then my friend Mara offered me laxatives so I could lose a couple of pounds really quickly, and I hate to admit it, but I jumped at the chance.

I know I shouldn't say this, but the laxatives were amazing, at least at first. I never felt bloated any more, and the dress fit perfectly at the prom. I just got hooked kind of fast. I'd take the stuff before I

went to bed, and I'd only feel uncomfortable for a short time each
morning. I felt great all day. And totally skinny.

After a few weeks, my parents found about five boxes of laxative tablets in my room, and they had a fit. First, I had to see my pediatrician, and then she recommended this guy, Dr. Anders.

THERAPIST: Was the therapy helpful?

SALLIE: Overall, it was okay, I guess. We talked a lot about college and
the end of high school. I did feel better having someone to talk to.

THERAPIST: How did the therapy end?

SALLIE: After a while, I just felt better, and then we met a few more times
before we stopped. Dr. Anders said I could always call him in the future if I wanted to talk. I didn't need to . . . until now, I guess.

THERAPIST: Did you think about calling him after the breakup with
Charlie?

SALLIE: I did talk to him twice a couple of weeks ago. He was the one
who recommended that I find a person to see up here. After we
talked a few times and I wasn't feeling better, he thought it would
be better to see someone face to face. I was crying so hard on the
phone, I think I freaked him out a little bit.

THERAPIST: Hmm, how did you feel when he recommended you find a
therapist locally?

SALLIE: (*Becomes tearful.*) I felt pretty upset. I know it is hard to get a
good sense of what is going on over the phone, but I was surprised
when he thought I was so messed up that I needed to see someone
else. I mean, he really knows me!

THERAPIST: Do you miss him?

SALLIE: I really do. No offense, Dr. Bender, but I don't know you at all. I
have to tell you all this history that he is already familiar with.

THERAPIST: It is doubly hard to start with someone new and to miss Dr.
Anders at the same time [*validating Sallie's experience rather than
taking offense*].

SALLIE: Yep . . . it is. Whatever . . . what other questions do you need to ask?

THERAPIST: Let's see . . . well, have you ever been on any psychiatric
medications?

SALLIE: No. Talking alone did the trick, at least in high school. Like I
said, until now I've been doing really well. My eating habits have
been really healthy for years now. The idea of taking laxatives again
is repulsive. At least, that's progress.

Even though I was scared of leaving home at first, I think it's been helpful to go to school away from home. I'm the oldest, so maybe it was extra hard to leave, but I think becoming more independent has been good for me.

THERAPIST: It is important progress that your eating has improved and that you no longer take laxatives.

You mentioned you are the oldest. How many siblngs do you have?

SALLIE: Just one. Tom is 6 years younger than me. He's 15.

THERAPIST: What is your relationship with him like?

SALLIE: Oh, good I guess. It's really fine.

THERAPIST: I definitely want to know more about Tom and your family, but I want to make sure that I get a chance to ask about your psychiatric and medical history. Have you ever been in a psychiatric hospital?

SALLIE: Actually, yes. Umm, I guess I forgot to mention that.

THERAPIST: When was that?

SALLIE: Well, after the prom when my parents found the laxatives, my pediatrician said that my lab data were dangerous, and she didn't trust me to stop the laxatives on my own. She sent me to the emergency room to get IV's and stuff, and the shrink that saw me at the hospital sent me to a psychiatric hospital. I'll never forgive him. It was the worst 10 days of my life.

Well, maybe it helped a tiny bit because I didn't use the laxatives ever again when I got out, but it's totally humiliating that I had to be locked up in a loony bin when I was in high school. I don't tell many people.

THERAPIST: Humiliated is how you feel, but it isn't the word that comes to mind for me. It sounds as though you were really struggling. What was the hospital's name?

SALLIE: Something-or-other Lodge.

THERAPIST: Were you in the hospital any other times?

SALLIE: No, just that once. I am not that much of a kook.

THERAPIST: Is it uncomfortable to talk about this sensitive time?

SALLIE: Sort of. I mean it's not something that I'm proud of.

THERAPIST: I am glad you felt comfortable enough to tell me about it. It sounds as though it was a difficult time, but you were able to take advantage of the help from the hospital and from Dr. Anders.

You overcame the crisis in high school. There's a good chance that the resilience you showed then will help you now, but we need to know more. [*Offering justifiable hope can be highly beneficial.*]

During this time in high school, did you have any thoughts of harming yourself?

SALLIE: Now and then . . .

THERAPIST: Were they passing thoughts or did you think of doing something?

SALLIE: Umm, mainly passing thoughts.

THERAPIST: What did you think about?

SALLIE: I just thought about what my funeral would be like . . . how many people would come. Actually, I would get depressed thinking about it because I didn't think any of my high school friends would even show up. I knew I would never do anything, though. My parents would have been too devastated.

THERAPIST: Did you ever think about how you might hurt yourself?

SALLIE: No, not specifically.

THERAPIST: Is there any other time in your life when you thought about suicide?

SALLIE: No, suicide has never really been an issue for me. Nowadays, I sometimes feel I just don't care about a lot of things, but I don't think I would go that far.

THERAPIST: Some people, under stressful circumstances, will attempt to relieve the emotional pain by cutting or burning themselves. Have you ever done this?

SALLIE: Oh, I just read an article about that for psych class. Nah, I'd never do that. Well, once I was sort of curious and I pricked myself once with a knife when I felt really angry, but it hurt, so I stopped.

THERAPIST: What stopped you?

SALLIE: I just imagined my parents finding out and shipping me off to the Lodge again. Plus, I don't like pain. I think I was just curious.

THERAPIST: How does it feel talking about this?

SALLIE: Okay, I guess. It was a long time ago. I've grown up a lot since then.

THERAPIST: You are doing a good job helping me get a sense of what this time was like for you. Has anyone else in your family ever been in a psychiatric hospital?

SALLIE: No.

THERAPIST: Does anyone in your family struggle with psychiatric difficulties, like anxiety, depression, or alcohol and substance abuse?

SALLIE: My mother's brother used to have a problem with alcohol, but he is okay now. He's been sober a number of years. My mother sometimes says she had the "baby blues" with me, but I don't really know what that means. She never went to a psychiatrist.

THERAPIST: Anyone in the family try to hurt himself in any way?

SALLIE: No, not as far as I know.

It's easy to swerve off course during the second session while you collect the past medical and psychiatric history. During Example 4.4, Sallie introduces a number of new topics that pique my interest (moving away to college, her brother Tom), but I stay focused, concentrating on Sallie's past outpatient and inpatient treatment, past trials of psychopharmacological medications, past suicidal behavior, and her family's psychiatric history. I "bookmark" the other topics for future discusssion.

For patients with prior therapy experience, I learn how long the prior treatment lasted and what the patient found helpful or not helpful. I try to pay special attention to how my new patient terminated with her previous therapist. Was she able to tolerate a planned good-bye, or did she disengage abruptly and without warning? People tend to replay their past. How my patient dealt with a former therapist may provide a clue for our future together.

If the previous therapy was a good experience, I acknowledge how difficult it is to start with someone new. Polite patients are unlikely to tell me this directly, but they may feel relieved and understood when I mention that switching therapists may be a difficult process.

As a psychiatrist, I collect a psychopharmacological history during this part of the consultation. In addition to learning which medications have been tried in the past, I ask how long each trial occurred, what was the maximum dose reached for each medication, which medications worked, and which side effects were experienced.

Even for therapists who do not prescribe medication, it is important to know whether your patient has ever taken any psychotropic drugs, such as antidepressants, lithium, benzodiazepines, or others. Learn which drugs have been tried and which were successful. Is she taking any now? Who prescribes them? Do not assume she isn't taking psychotropic medications if she isn't seeing a psychiatrist. Many primary care doctors will prescribe antidepressants, such as fluoxetine, or antianxiety medications, such as clonazepam or alprazolam.

For past psychiatric hospitalizations, I learn the basic details about the admissions (when and where they occurred, how long they lasted, whether any medications were tried during the admissions, and the details of the postinpatient followup). At this time, Sallie remains very vague about the details of her psychiatric admission during high school. As we continue to work together and Sallie begins to trust me, I hope to learn more about this stressful time. I could also obtain her inpatient psychiatric records for my files. This early in the consultation it is normal to have only an outline of the patient's history, like a coloring book that hasn't been filled in yet.

As prior suicidal behavior is one of the strongest predictors of future attempts, it is essential to clarify past suicidal history, including specific thoughts and actions the patient has had about self-harm throughout her life. For any suicidal thoughts, I ask for a detailed account of any actions that occurred as well. For instance, if she had a fleeting plan of overdosing when she was a teenager, did she just think about it, or did she collect pills, count them out, and hold them in her hand?

Questions about self-mutilatory behavior can follow the questions about suicide. For any repetitive self-injurious act, it is important to elicit details about the symptom. For example: For cutting, I ask where and how deeply the patient cuts herself, how often she does it, and what triggers the activity. For medical reasons, it is useful to know what instrument she uses to hurt herself, and if she has ever required medical attention for this behavior. If the patient is using unclean implements, I ask about her most recent tetanus booster, as it needs to be updated every 10 years. (For more help on how to respond to self-destructive behavior and to an actively suicidal patient, please see Chapter 9.)

I also gather information on medical history, medications, and allergies during this second session.

EXAMPLE 4.5

Collecting a personal and family medical history

THERAPIST: We need to review your medical history. Do you have any major medical problems?

SALLIE: No.

THERAPIST: Have you ever been in a medical hospital overnight for any reason?

SALLIE: Oh, yeah, when I was 10 I had an infection in my hand, and I needed to be hospitalized for IV antibiotics.

THERAPIST: How did it feel to be hospitalized overnight at such a young age?

SALLIE: It was scary, but it was only a few days, so it wasn't too horrible.

THERAPIST: Do you have any residual problems with your hand?

SALLIE: No, it is okay, luckily.

THERAPIST: Any other medical problems as a child? Any other major infections, surgeries, broken bones?

SALLIE: Let me think. No other infections. No surgeries. Only a broken wrist once. Oh, yes, I had tubes in my ear when I was baby because I had so many ear infections, but I don't remember much about that, obviously. I do remember my mother saying that I was a trouper and never complained about all my doctor's visits. [*Sallie is beginning to follow the therapist's lead, not only stating the facts, but also trying to remember how the incident affected her.*]

THERAPIST: Any other recurrent chronic medical problems with any part of your body? Any problems with asthma? Any stomach problems?

SALLIE: No. No.

THERAPIST: Have you ever had head trauma where you lost consciousness?

SALLIE: I don't think so, but I fainted once when I was really tired and standing up too long on a really hot day.

THERAPIST: Did you hit your head?

SALLIE: No. My dad caught me as I went down.

THERAPIST: Ever have any seizures?

SALLIE: Umm, I don't think so, I'd know if I had that, right?

THERAPIST: (*Nods.*) When is the last time you had a physical exam? Do you have any current physical symptoms that are bothering you?

SALLIE: Oh, I had a physical about 6 months ago. Everything was fine.

THERAPIST: Who is your primary care physician?

SALLIE: Well, I got my physical at school from a doctor at the student health services. Her name was Dr. Newman, but at home my doctor is Dr. Karen.

THERAPIST: Do you have any current physical symptoms that are bothering you? (*repeating the question because Sallie did not answer it the first time around*)

SALLIE: I have been feeling very tired lately. But I figured that it was just because I am overwhelmed with this whole Charlie incident.

THERAPIST: Did the tiredness start before or after you had your physical 6 months ago?

SALLIE: Oh, it's relatively recent; I've only had it about 2 months now.

THERAPIST: The tiredness may be related to the breakup with Charlie, but there are also a number of medical conditions that can cause fatigue. It may be worth making an appointment with Dr. Newman to make sure that you don't have any other medical reason to be so tired.

SALLIE: Okay.

THERAPIST: Have you been taking any medications, prescribed or over-the-counter?

SALLIE: I take ibuprofen every month with my period, and vitamins, but that's it.

THERAPIST: Which vitamins?

SALLIE: Umm, I take a vitamin C supplement and a multivitamin.

THERAPIST: Are you allergic to any medicines?

SALLIE: Maybe penicillin. I think I get a rash from that.

THERAPIST: Are you currently sexually active?

SALLIE: Umm, yes . . . at least I was before Charlie and I broke up.

THERAPIST: What did you use for contraception?

SALLIE: Oh, yeah, I'm also on the pill.

THERAPIST: Oh, okay. Did you know Charlie's HIV status?

SALLIE: Umm, no. But I'm sure he's fine.

THERAPIST: Hmmm . . . I wouldn't be doing my job if I didn't ask how you were protecting yourself from sexually transmitted diseases with the pill.

SALLIE: Oh, I think Charlie was safe. He didn't sleep around a lot.

THERAPIST: You know, it really is a very difficult situation nowadays to have to be so careful during sex, but the safest approach is for you to be medically checked for HIV or other sexually transmitted diseases.

SALLIE: Oh, I don't think that's necessary. I knew Charlie for a while before we went out. He's clean.

THERAPIST: I am glad you did think about it. I feel a bit in a bind, because I think your health is awfully important, but I also don't think it is my role as your therapist to act as the sex police. [*I make a mental note to bring this up again if the opportunity presents itself, for instance, if Sallie starts a new relationship.*]

SALLIE: Yeah, I hear your point, but I really think I was safe enough here.

THERAPIST: Do your parents have any medical problems?

SALLIE: No. They are pretty healthy overall. My dad has some arthritis from some old sports injuries, but otherwise they're doing pretty well. They like sports and do a lot of outdoor activities together.

THERAPIST: And your brother?

SALLIE: He has a history of stomach problems, but he's better now.

THERAPIST: What kind of stomach problems?

SALLIE: He used to have a lot of trouble with chronic stomach pain and diarrhea, but he's recovered now.

THERAPIST: I've asked you a lot of questions today, and I am beginning to get a good overview. How has it felt for you?

SALLIE: It is weird to think about the psych hospitalization during high school. I don't usually talk about that, but the rest was okay.

THERAPIST: Well, I appreciate you being so open with me about your experience. Next week, we'll cover some more of my questions, and we'll be closer to making a treatment plan.

SALLIE: Oh, good. I really want to get back to talking about Charlie.

THERAPIST: We still have about 10 minutes today. Could you fill me in? What would you like to tell me?

A thorough medical history should cover Sallie's current physical health as well as her personal and family medical history. During this part of the consultation, I always ask specifically about a history of significant or repeated head trauma with loss of consciousness. With significant head injury, a patient is at risk for cognitive impairment, seizures, and emotional lability. A history of such events added to current neurological impairment may warrant further evaluation by a neurologist or by a psychiatrist who is familiar with the behavioral manifestations of brain damage.

It's often not easy to gather a sexual history. First, I may not know whether my new patient is straight, gay, or bisexual, and to be an effective therapist I have to be ready to accept any of these orientations. During medical school at the University of California, San Francisco, I was taught to ask about sexuality with two questions: "Are you sexually active?" followed by "With men, women, or both?" While this approach is helpful for the gay or bisexual patient, it is often embarrassing for the straight, conservative patient. Nowadays, I use the first part of the question and then follow the patient's lead. I try not to assume that the patient's partner will be of the opposite sex until I hear this fact explicitly. I think this more cautious approach is more sensitive than the medical school method, although it may not be as absolutely politically correct.

A therapist is often in the unenviable position of hearing about a patient's poor judgment that puts her at physical or emotional risk. In Sallie's case, she had put herself at risk with her unsafe sex with Charlie. As a health practitioner, it is not responsible to ignore your patient's risky behavior, but a righteous directive stance is unlikely to promote change. During my first months as a psychotherapist, I didn't know how to approach these sensitive issues in a therapeutic way. I spent many uncomfortable sessions inwardly screaming "STOP IT!" while I listened to patients describe their numerous sexual escapades without a condom, their experimentation with powerful hallucinogens, or their driving recklessly 60 miles an hour down a side street without a seatbelt.

If preaching worked, I'd use it, but the last thing any patient needs is another directive, unempathic person in her life. While it can be terrifying to worry about your patients' safety, the only way she will ultimately change her behavior is by overcoming her inner resistance to protecting herself. Usually, this process takes time and occurs as the therapy slowly evolves. Meanwhile, your job is to acknowledge that the behavior is dangerous but to avoid becoming a nag. The strategy outlined in Example 4.5 is balanced, because it provides education and understanding without a domineering attitude. Our goal as therapists is to guide deftly but not to pretend that we have control.

Even if the patient doesn't protest about spending the majority of the session relating her medical and psychiatric history, I leave about 10–15 minutes at the end of the session to talk about the primary difficulty that brought her to treatment. The patient will appreciate that I haven't forgotten her main concerns, and this will also be my opportunity to arrange for the third session.

EXAMPLE 4.6

Closing the second session

THERAPIST: Well, I appreciate your being so open with me about your experience. Next week we'll cover some more questions, and we'll be closer to making a treatment plan.

SALLIE: Oh, good. I really want to get back to talking about Charlie.

THERAPIST: We still have about 10 minutes today. Could you fill me in? What would you like to tell me?

SALLIE: Umm, I don't know. What should I do this week to get through it? When do you think I'll feel better?

THERAPIST: What has helped you get through it so far?

SALLIE: Distraction works the best, I guess. But, how long will this therapy take to work? Last time with Dr. Anders I was a little upset but nothing like this. How long do you think it will take for me to feel better?

THERAPIST: I can understand it might be difficult to be patient because you have been feeling bad for so long. I wish I could say some words that could take all your pain away, but unfortunately it isn't that simple. If it were easy to fix, you wouldn't even be seeing me in the first place. You would have figured this thing out by yourself long ago. I think we both need to keep working on this together.

SALLIE: Oh, okay. I wish it could be faster too, but if this is the way it has to be, I'll just manage as best I can.

THERAPIST: Which distractions work best?

SALLIE: Movies, running—even studying sometimes. (*Laughs.*)

THERAPIST: Sounds good. Until next week . . .

SALLIE: Yeah, I'll see you then.

The consultation is well on its way. Sallie is beginning to trust me, and I am slowly getting an outline of her story, both present and past.

> **Review of mnemonic for depression:** SIGECAPS—sleep, interest, guilt, energy, concentration, appetite, psychomotor, suicide
>
> **Key words:** anorexia nervosa, bulimia, diagnosis, dysphoria, eating disorders, evaluation, family history, major depression, medical history, neurovegetative symptoms, psychiatric history, psychotherapy, safety, safe sex, self-harm, sexually transmitted diseases, suicide, therapeutic alliance

SAMPLE CONSULTATION QUESTIONNAIRE

To the patient:

The information in this questionnaire will help me understand your situation. When added to our meetings together, it will help us find an effective approach to the problems that we shall be considering together. Your replies will be held in confidence as required by law.

Please add any information that you believe might be relevant, using the reverse sides of pages if necessary.

Name _____ Date _____

Date of birth _____

Address _____

Telephone numbers: Home _____
                                 Work _____

Occupation _____

Social Security Number _____

Who referred you to me? _____

Health insurance _____ Group _____
Policy _____

Emergency contact information:
Name _____
Address _____
Phone number _____

What is the main concern that led you to consult me? _____
_____
_____

MEDICAL HISTORY

Allergies

Are you allergic to any medicines? Yes _____ No _____
If yes, please list:

Are you allergic to other substances? Yes _____ No _____
If yes, which ones?

What types of allergic reactions have you had?

Medical Illnesses

Have you had any illnesses in the past? Yes _____ No _____
If yes, which ones?

Do you have any illnesses at present? Yes _____ No _____
If yes, which are they?

Date of your most recent physical examination _____

Name of your physician _____
Address _____
Telephone number _____

Do you authorize me to communicate with your physician? Yes _____ No _____

Surgical Conditions

Have you had surgical operations or injuries? Yes _____ No _____

If yes, what were they and when did you have them?

Date of your most recent tetanus booster _____

Have you ever had a head injury? Yes _____ No _____

Did you lose consciousness? Yes _____ No _____

When did this happen?

How did it occur?

Have you ever had seizures? Yes _____ No _____
If so, what are they like?

PSYCHIATRIC HISTORY
Hospitalizations

Have you ever been hospitalized for a psychiatric disorder? Yes _____ No _____
If yes, what was the disorder, which hospital(s), and what were the dates?

Outpatient Psychiatric Treatment

Have you ever had out-of-hospital treatment for a psychiatric disorder?
Yes _____ No _____
If yes, what was the disorder?

When and where did you receive the treatment?

What type of treatment was it (e.g., psychotherapy, medication, behavior therapy, others)?

Name of your former therapist _____
Address _____
Telephone number _____
Do you authorize me to communicate with him/her? Yes ____ No ____

MEDICATION HISTORY

Which medications are you taking now (medical or psychiatric)?

Drug   Dose   Frequency   Prescribing physician

_____

_____

_____

_____

Which medications have you taken in the past?

Drug   Date   Reason for discontinuing

_____

_____

_____

_____

Do you use nonprescription medications? Yes ____ No ____
If yes, which ones?

Do you or have you used recreational or illegal drugs? Yes ____ No ____
If yes, which drugs and how much?

Do you drink alcohol? Yes ____ No ____
Have you ever tried to cut down on how much you drink? Yes ____ No ____
Are you annoyed at comments about your drinking? Yes ____ No ____
Have you felt guilty about anything resulting from your drinking? Yes ____ No ____
Do you feel better if you have a drink early in the day? Yes ____ No ____
Do you smoke? Yes ____ No ____
If yes, what and how much?

Any uses of nonsmoking forms of tobacco? Yes ____ No ____
If yes, which?

Beverages with caffeine:

(Circle those that apply)

Coffee or tea _____ cups per day

Colas _____ cans per day

FAMILY PSYCHIATRIC HISTORY

Has anyone in your family ever had a psychiatric disorder? Yes _____ No _____
Have any of the following family members had psychiatric disorders (including depression, mania, schizophrenia, drug or alcohol abuse, obsessive–compulsive disorder, panic disorder, phobias, suicide)? Please indicate diagnosis and the name of the individual.

Your sons or daughters _____
Father _____
Mother _____
Brothers _____
Sisters _____
Maternal grandparents _____
Paternal grandparents _____
Uncles/aunts/cousins _____

Marital Status
Single _____ Married _____ Widowed _____ Divorced _____
If married, date of wedding _____
    Husband's/wife's date of birth _____
    Occupation of husband/wife _____

If widowed, date of spouse's death _____
    Cause of death _____
If separated/divorced, date _____
    Reason _____
Children
Name   Date of birth

_____   _____
_____   _____
_____   _____
_____   _____

Do you engage in safe sex?   Always   Sometimes   Never
Do you have any sexual concerns? Yes _____ No _____
Which form(s) of birth control do you use? _____
Others currently living in your household and their relationship to you
Name   Relationship

_____   _____
_____   _____
_____   _____
_____   _____
_____   _____

FAMILY MEDICAL HISTORY

Mother's name _____ Age _____
    If deceased, date and cause of death _____
    Serious illnesses _____
Father's name _____ Age _____
    If deceased, date and cause of death _____
    Serious illnesses _____

Brothers and sisters
Name   Serious Illnesses

_____   _____

_____   _____

_____   _____

_____   _____

BRIEF REVIEW OF SYSTEMS

SYMPTOM OR PROBLEM—Circle all that apply. If circled, please describe in more detail and make a note of the date it began.

- Decreased vision/eye pain
- Wear eyeglasses/contacts
- Dizziness/vertigo
- Earaches/buzzing or other sounds
- Decreased hearing
- Difficulty swallowing
- Chest pain
- Shortness of breath
- Decreased energy
- Difficulty concentrating/distractibility
- Difficulties with organization
- Impulsivity
- Cough/asthma
- Abdominal pain
- Menstrual/reproductive problems or infections
- Eating problems
- Decreased appetite
- Using laxatives, diuretics, or diet pills to lose weight
- Nausea/vomiting/diarrhea
- Weight loss/gain
- Bloody or black stools
- Blood in urine
- Frequent or severe headaches
- Convulsions or seizures
- Self-induced vomiting with or without ipecac
- Depression
- Anxiety/panic attacks
- Avoidance of public places in order to avoid panic attacks
- Sleep difficulty
- Decreased motivation
- Racing thoughts
- Suicidal thoughts/fears
- Suicidal wishes/plans/attempts
- Homicidal thoughts/wishes
- Homicidal plans/violent acts
- Seeing things that other people don't see
- Hearing things that other people don't hear
- Legal history—trouble with the law
- Loneliness/isolation

- Repetitive unwanted thoughts or actions
- Hopelessness/guilt
- Checking things multiple times to make sure they are in place
- Washing things multiple times to make sure they are clean
- Nightmares
- Flashbacks

Does your primary care physician know about the symptoms you have circled?
Yes _____ No _____

Have you ever been exposed to abuse? Yes _____ No _____
    Physical _____
    Sexual _____
    Emotional _____
Who was involved?

Are you distressed about any aspect of your appearance? Yes _____ No _____

Have you ever donated blood? Yes _____ No _____
If you have, when was the most recent donation?

EDUCATIONAL HISTORY

Name of School/Location	Dates
Elementary	
Secondary	
College	
Postgraduate	

Have you had any history of difficulties at school? Yes _____ No _____
If yes, please describe:

OCCUPATIONAL HISTORY

Dates	Job Titles	Exposure to Dangerous Substances

Military Service _____

Have you had any history of difficulties at work? Yes _____ No _____
If yes, please explain.

Have you had any problems with the law? Yes _____ No _____
If yes, please explain.

DEVELOPMENTAL HISTORY

Was your mother exposed to stresses, drugs, or dangerous substances while pregnant with you? Yes ____ No ____
If yes, what were they?

Were there any difficulties with your birth? Yes ____ No ____
If yes, what were they?

Did you have any difficulties in your physical development? Yes ____ No ____
If yes, what were they?

Have you had any recent stresses or relevant stresses in the past?
Yes ____ No ____
If yes, please list them.

ADAPTIVE HISTORY

Which stresses have you overcome in the past?

How did you do it?

What was the best period of your life?

What are your personal strengths?

Please sign this questionnaire.

_____

5

Collecting a Psychosocial History and Screening for Common Psychological Disorders

To facilitate arrival at an accurate diagnosis and to formulate an effective treatment plan, it is important to collect relevant history concerning the patient's childhood and later development as well as information about substance abuse, anxiety disorders, psychosis, mania, and self-injurious behavior.

THE BEGINNING OF THE THIRD SESSION

I don't especially like psychiatric consultations. Ongoing treatment is a different story. It's a special privilege to work over time with a patient on her most pressing and private concerns. Consultations, in contrast, are a bit of a slog because I need to collect so much information in a short amount of time. Part of me has always wanted to skip the consultation process altogether, but I'm now resigned that a thorough evaluation is actually the best way to start an effective psychotherapy. Thankfully, once I've finished asking the questions reviewed in this chapter, I'm more than halfway done.

A quick review of Sallie's first and second visits: During Session 1, I focused on Sallie's main concern and only directed the interview to assess suicidality and safety, the most urgent parts of the mental status examination—unless the patient is homicidal or is openly psychotic. (For an example of a more complete mental status examination, see the sample consultation summary at the end of this chapter.) During Session 2, I used a more structured approach and asked Sallie about her current depressive symptoms and her past psychiatric and medical history. While I've tried many different ways to organize the first two sessions, I like this approach the best. It balances the need to establish a therapeutic alliance with the need to gather pertinent clinical information.

During Session 3, my first round of questions will focus on Sallie's developmental history. Before the meeting, I review the information I already have and make a special notation of the questions I still need to cover. Using the strategy outlined in Example 4.1, I gently interrupt Sallie after she talks freely for the first 10 minutes of the session, leading with an empathic statement as I redirect the conversation. (For example: "This has really been a tough time. While I also want to hear how you have been feeling during the last week, I would like to use this session and the next one if necessary to finish collecting the information I need to plan an effective treatment.")

COLLECTING A DEVELOPMENTAL HISTORY

When eliciting a developmental history, I am guided by Freud's basic adage that a person is emotionally stable when she has succeeded in both love and work. For a child, immediate family and school serve as the first love and the first work experiences. Over time, I'll learn about each member of the Gane family and paint a mental picture of Sallie interacting with her parents and brother. As children mature, they form significant relationships with their peers, so I'll also focus on Sallie's past and current friendships and romantic relationships. As the ability to make and keep friends is an important developmental step, the lack of friends during latency can be a clue to a profound sense of isolation.

For a school history, I'll eventually want to know about Sallie's school experience at different ages, including preschool, latency (elementary school), adolescence, and beyond. Persistent profound difficulties in school may signal an unrecognized diagnosis of attention-deficit/hyperactivity disorder or a learning disability.

As I construct an impression of Sallie's life, I'll listen for significant childhood life events, especially those that can have a profound impact on a child: a relative's or friend's death, a mother's miscarriage, a move across the country or even to another school district, a divorce, or an illness suffered either by the patient or by someone close to her. The patient's age at the time of the event is important. A 4-year-old, for instance, will process a family crisis very differently than will a 10-year-old.

Positive memories are equally important. To have a clear picture of Sallie's development, I'll eventually want to know some of her favorite activities as a child, her natural talents, and what she wanted to be when she grew up.

As I gather all of this information, I'll be trying to understand why Sallie is currently having trouble finding contentment in her life. Interestingly enough, difficulties in work and love are often intertwined.

There are two main strategies a therapist can use to collect a developmental history, each with its own set of pros and cons. With a sequential approach, the therapist asks about the patient's past very slowly, starting with her birth and then gradually advancing up the developmental ladder until the present.

With the sequential approach, my knowledge of Sallie's upbringing would be extraordinarily detailed, but there may be a therapeutic cost. In order to gather so much information, I'll have to be fairly directive, and I may miss opportunities to discuss any emotionally pertinent topics in more detail. If the process becomes prolonged, Sallie may feel frustrated that her primary concern, Charlie, is not being addressed.

I prefer to collect a developmental history by asking questions about the patient's past that specifically relate to her present concern. This method is illustrated in Example 5.1.

EXAMPLE 5.1

Obtaining a developmental history by following the patient's lead

SALLIE: I just feel so punk about Charlie and the breakup. (*Sniffles.*)

THERAPIST: (*Waits in silence for Sallie to continue.*)

SALLIE: I don't even know what to say anymore.

THERAPIST: You have mentioned before that the relationship with Charlie felt very different from your relationships with other boyfriends. Could you tell me more about that?

SALLIE: Yeah, sure. Well, my first boyfriend's name was Larry. We went out for 3 months during my freshman year of college. He was very sweet, just very boring.

THERAPIST: What made him boring?

SALLIE: It's weird. The features that attracted me to him in the first place were also the reasons I couldn't stand him by the end.

THERAPIST: What were those features?

SALLIE: Well, at first I just thought he was the best. He brought me flowers all the time. I think he looked up to me. I mean, he had me on—

What do you call it?—oh, yeah, a pedestal. Basically, Larry thought I was perfect, and who was I to disagree? (*Grins.*) But he let me boss him around. That wasn't so good, I think.

THERAPIST: Can you give me some examples?

SALLIE: I don't know. . . .

THERAPIST: (*Waits quietly with an interested look.*)

SALLIE: Well, for instance, if I wanted to go out to dinner, we went out to dinner. If I wanted to go shopping, we went shopping. At first, I loved the fact that I always got my way, but then (I hate to say this, but I think it's true) . . . I started taking advantage. I think I was sort of pushy, and he never stood up for himself. This sounds horrible, but I think I got bored.

THERAPIST: How did the relationship end?

SALLIE: Umm, well, I sort of lied to break it off. I told Larry that I needed to devote time to my studies, and I couldn't afford to be distracted with a boyfriend. Then, I stopped answering his calls. Eventually, he got the message.

THERAPIST: What was that like for you?

SALLIE: I feel guilty that I didn't feel more upset. Maybe I am a hardhearted person, I don't know. But, after I broke it off, I felt 10 pounds lighter. Even though Larry was *so* nice to me, he made me feel squished.

THERAPIST: And the second boyfriend?

SALLIE: Oh, Alec . . . well, he was a premed student. When we first met, he was majoring in biochemistry. It looked like he had goals other than focusing on me, and I liked that.

But the strangest thing happened. After we went out for a few months, he started acting just like Larry. It was bizarre. He had been so independent, and then, all of a sudden, he was constantly catering to me. I don't really know how it happened, but once I knew I had the upper hand, I lost interest again.

See, this is why Charlie is such a find. He's interesting and always has an opinion that he is willing to defend, even if I disagree with it. Life with him was never boring. I sometimes fantasized about marrying him. . . . (*Looks down abruptly and eyes well up with tears.*)

THERAPIST: This breakup was so painful because you felt that you had found someone very special?

SALLIE: That's true.

THERAPIST: How did you imagine marriage to Charlie would be?

SALLIE: Fun. New adventures together all the time. Taking chances. Not like my parents' marriage.

THERAPIST: Could you tell me more about your parents' relationship?

SALLIE: Why? There is nothing wrong with them. (*Looks annoyed.*)

THERAPIST: [*I reword the question to correct Sallie's impression that I was criticizing her parents' relationship.*] Well, when searching for a partner, it is impossible not to be affected by your experience of your parent's relationship. What is their marriage like?

SALLIE: Oh, it's fine.

THERAPIST: What is fine about it? How do they interact?

SALLIE: Well, they basically get along. But they are very different.

THERAPIST: How are they different?

SALLIE: Well, my mom has always reminded me of a hummingbird. She never stops moving; she has so much energy. When I was growing up, all my friends would always want to come over to my house because my mom was the most fun. She's very cutting edge. We used to read the fashion magazines together when I was in high school. Did I tell you? I even won "best dressed" in high school, but she was the one that really deserved the award.

THERAPIST: Does she work outside of the home as well?

SALLIE: She's a real estate agent part time. She likes it, but it isn't her dream job. She talks a lot about starting her own business, but she wants to wait until my brother is more healthy and in college.

She is really supportive of me though. She loves that I'm studying economics. She always says it will prepare me to do whatever I want when I graduate.

THERAPIST: You mentioned that she is very different from your dad. Can you tell me more?

SALLIE: Well, my dad is sort of quiet. He makes a lot of jokes, but he was always the calm influence at home. My mom flits around nonstop, and my dad is happy to sit in one place and read or watch TV. I think they are good for each other in this way, but they are very different.

THERAPIST: What does your dad do for a living?

SALLIE: He's a manager of an electronics store. He likes gadgets, and he's good with people, but once he's home he just wants to be with us.

He's my reading buddy, because we'll read the same stuff and then talk it over. I love that.

THERAPIST: What are your parents like together?

SALLIE: Cute, I guess. But they bicker a lot, too. My Mom always wants things a certain way, so they tend to get into arguments.

THERAPIST: What happens during a typical argument? [*I use the word argument to describe the interaction, as Sallie did.*]

SALLIE: If my mother wants to have a dinner party and my dad just wants a quiet evening at home, they yell about it for at least half an hour, sometimes longer. It's amazing how these little disagreements can blow out of proportion.

THERAPIST: How do you feel when you listen to it?

SALLIE: Annoyed. It's stupid, but it's just the way they do things.

THERAPIST: How does it usually end?

SALLIE: Oh, it usually ends the same way. My dad gets sick of arguing and my mom gets her way. I think it's strange that he doesn't get resentful. I would if I were giving in as much as he does, but he tells us, "I didn't realize how important this was to your mother, so we will do it her way." Then, they are all lovey-dovey—until the next fight, that is.

THERAPIST: How long has this type of fighting been part of their relationship?

SALLIE: Umm, as long as I can remember, but maybe it has gotten more frequent over the last few years.

When I follow Sallie's associations and ask detailed questions, our discussion about her submissive former boyfriends leads naturally into a conversation about her parents. She describes situations and scenes with specifics and emotions, and her stories are inherently interesting.

Example 5.1 also illustrates some techniques that help Sallie talk more specifically when she starts speaking in generalities and vague statements. When Sallie worries that my interest in her parent's marriage is a surreptitious dig for psychopathology, I openly describe the intent behind my line of questioning: "When searching for a partner, it is impossible not to be affected by your experience of your parents' relationship. What is their marriage like?" When she describes her parents' marriage as "fine," I ask for more details: "What is fine about it?"

In this interview, I use the question "What was that like for you?" after Sallie describes her breakup with Larry. For a patient who has a difficult time describing her emotions, this query is less threatening than the ubiquitous "How did that feel"? With "What was that like for you?" the patient can choose to answer with either cognition or emotion, whichever feels more accessible. As the therapy progresses and the patient is more comfortable expressing her emotions, I might focus more exclusively on affect, but at this point my main goal is to facilitate the conversation and the therapeutic alliance.

Since this second history-taking approach requires that I follow the patient's associations, rather than direct the collection of data, it takes more time to learn about Sallie's early childhood. Some topics (grade school, best friend, puberty) may not be covered until the therapy is well underway, so I keep a running mental list of the subjects I'll ask about when the appropriate time presents itself. Another option is to present Sallie with our questionnaire (at the end of Chapter 4) at the end of the first session to obtain some background, and then use Example 5.1's method to fill in the details over time.

FILLING IN THE GAPS:
COMPLETING A REVIEW OF SYSTEMS

Before the consultation concludes, I need to make sure that I have a comprehensive understanding of Sallie's difficulties. In medicine, an internist runs through a list of questions related to the main physiological systems in the body (such as cardiovascular and gastrointestinal) to see if her patient has any symptoms that she did not mention spontaneously. This is called a review of systems. In psychotherapy, a clinician needs to complete an analagous review to uncover pertinent psychological symptoms.

SCREENING FOR SUBSTANCE ABUSE

When considering a patient for psychotherapy, ruling out active addictive behavior is a crucial part of the consultation process, especially as most substance abusers rarely disclose their addictive behavior spontaneously during the first few interviews. If my new patient is actively abusing alcohol or drugs, my treatment approach needs to be modified, as outlined in Chapter 12, or the therapy has the potential to be destructive.

Unless a psychotherapy patient with an active drug problem is also in concurrent intensive substance abuse treatment, psychodynamic treatment may actually exacerbate the patient's substance abuse. The normal process of insight-oriented dynamic psychotherapy, uncovering and discussing emotionally laden topics, may be unbearable to a substance abuser unless she uses her drug of choice to numb herself against overwhelming affect. With this knowledge, some therapists won't even treat a substance abuser with psychotherapy until they have a number of months of sobriety under their belt.

For these reasons, I start my psychological review of systems by screening for substance abuse. Of course, how I ask these sensitive questions will affect the truthfulness of my patient's responses. Some possible approaches follow.

EXAMPLE 5.2

Three strategies to assess substance abuse during the consultation

THERAPIST: Now, as part of your medical history, when you drink socially, what is your drink of choice?

SALLIE: Beer mainly. Just on weekends.

THERAPIST: How many can you hold down? Can you hold down a six-pack?

SALLIE: At the very end of high school, around the time I was using the laxatives, I liked to drink, but everybody was doing it. By senior year, I could drink as much as my guy friends without passing out!

THERAPIST: Could you hold down more than a six-pack?

SALLIE: Nah, but almost. Nowadays, I feel dizzy after just one beer. I guess I've turned into a lightweight. (*Chuckles.*)

THERAPIST: Have you ever experimented with any other drugs?

SALLIE: Just marijuana.

THERAPIST: When is the last time you used it?

SALLIE: Oh, maybe 2 months ago. I only use it at parties. I don't buy it.

THERAPIST: How often do you tend to use it?

SALLIE: Oh, not often. Maybe every few months or so. I'm not into that stuff.

THERAPIST: I have a list of drugs I review with every patient. Bear with me as I go through it with you, but, as all of these drugs can affect mood, I need to know if you have ever tried them. Have you ever used cocaine or heroin?

SALLIE: No, I never tried those.

THERAPIST: Have you ever used antianxiety medications—either by prescription by a doctor or by buying them on the street, medications like Valium, Xanax, or Klonopin?

SALLIE: Actually, my roommate takes Klonopin for panic attacks and she gave me one last week when I couldn't sleep, but I didn't like the way it made me feel.

THERAPIST: Have you ever used uppers or downers?

SALLIE: No, no way.

THERAPIST: Sometimes people in college try hallucinogens like LSD or mushrooms. Have you?

SALLIE: I almost did it once at a party, but then I got scared. I'm pretty conservative actually, compared to some people I know. I'm not into drugs.

THERAPIST: I'm not asking these questions because I think you are into drugs, but a lot of people your age use substances to drown their sorrows when they are having a tough time. Has that been part of your experience?

SALLIE: No, I'm more of an ice cream-oholic. Give me a pint of cookies and cream anytime. If I'm really upset, I'll eat the whole carton.

Taking an accurate substance abuse history requires some clinical finesse because a patient is likely to report minimal use no matter what her actual intake. For this reason, we recommend asking about alcohol and drug use in three different ways, as illustrated in Example 5.2.

First, I assume that my patient does drink socially, as most people do, and I ask about her "drink of choice." Patients who drink heavily may minimize their use, but they are unlikely to deny all intake. With this question, I also identify the true teetotalers who avoid any alcohol intake no matter what the occasion. While patients who abstain from alcohol completely are unlikely to have a current substance abuse problem, further questioning may reveal either a past personal or family history of substance abuse.

Second, after asking about the drink of choice, I learn about my patient's alcohol tolerance. When talking with Sallie, my first guesstimate of her alcohol use ("a six-pack?") is purposely high; she's more likely to confess her actual intake if it's lower than my questioned estimate. While Sallie's current alcohol intake is moderate, her drinking in high school did sound worrisome. Any woman of average height and weight who can manage more than two or three beers at a sitting has a higher than normal tolerance, which often reflects a sign of more frequent alcohol intake. While tolerance is not synonymous with addiction, it is a potential clue.

I use my questions about alcohol to transition to a substance abuse history. Even if my patient has only experimented with marijuana, I'll ask briefly about all other drugs as well. If she has ever tried a particular substance, I'll learn how long she has been using it, how much, and how often. For certain drugs such as cocaine and heroin, the method of use (snorted, smoked, or injected) is also relevant.

As a third strategy to unmask surreptitious addiction, I refer to substance use as a coping mechanism for emotional pain: "Have you ever tried to drown your sorrows or to comfort yourself with alcohol or drugs?" Understanding that substance use may be my patient's last-ditch effort to cope with a difficult situation might facilitate a more honest intake report.

Finally, it can be useful to finish this part of the interview with the CAGE questionnaire, a short, valid, reliable, and nonconfrontational survey that screens for addiction. The CAGE questionnaire allows any health practitioner to screen for substance abuse during a brief office visit. It's easy to learn and easy to remember.

Each letter in the acronym stands for a question about substance use. While the CAGE questionnaire was originally created to study alcohol use, to maximize the bang for my buck I ask about all possible addictive substances simultaneously. The questions are as follows: C: Have you ever in your life tried to CUT DOWN on your drinking (or drug use?) If so, when? A: Have people ever ANNOYED you by criticizing your drinking (or drug use)? (A useful additional question: Has anyone ever been ANNOYED at you because of your alcohol or drug use?) G: Have you ever felt bad or GUILTY about your drinking (or drug use)? What have you done under the influence? E: Have you ever had a drink (or drug) first thing in the morning to steady your nerves or to get rid of a hangover? (EYE-OPENER) Research has shown that two positive answers to the CAGE questionnaire will identify 90% of substance abusers, regardless of the patient's reported use.

For simplicity's sake, we've spared Sallie a current substance abuse problem. Her therapy won't need the specialized addiction approach. To illustrate the use of the CAGE with an active substance abuser, we'll introduce a second fictional patient, Anthony Lee, in Example 5.3. Mr. Lee is a 35-year-old business consultant who will reappear in Chapter 12 to help us demonstrate the special clinical issues involved in psychotherapy with a substance abuser.

EXAMPLE 5.3

Assessing substance abuse using the CAGE questionnaire

Midway into the third session of the consultation with Anthony, I start to ask my questions about substance abuse. After Anthony admits to social use of alcohol and denies all drug use, I move on to the CAGE questionnaire.

THERAPIST: I have four questions about substance use that I ask every new patient during a consultation. It may feel a bit strange to hear these questions since you have just told me you only drink on weekends, but I do think they are important to review. First, have you ever in your life tried to cut down on your alcohol or drug use?

ANTHONY: Well, not really. Nowadays, I make sure I only drink a few beers a night at most. Maybe a little more on the weekends. [*This counts as a YES = C+*]

THERAPIST: Have you ever been annoyed by other people criticizing your drinking or drug use?

ANTHONY: Dr. Bender, I don't use any drugs. A couple of girlfriends have nagged me about my drinking, but that is because they come from such a puritanical background. My family has a high tolerance for alcohol, and my work has never suffered from my socializing on the weekend. [*This also counts as a YES = C+ A+*]

THERAPIST: Have you ever felt guilty about your drinking or any past drug use?

ANTHONY: Not really . . .

THERAPIST: (*Quietly waits.*)

ANTHONY: Well, maybe just a tad, but not really. Even if I feel guilty easily, I don't think my drinking is anything to worry about. [*C+ A+ G+*]

THERAPIST: Have you ever used any drug or alcohol in the morning to help you steady your nerves or to alleviate a hangover?

ANTHONY: Never. I don't drink in the mornings. Ever. [*This counts as a NO = E−*]

With three positive responses on the CAGE questionnaire, Anthony qualifies as an active substance abuser. In Chapter 12, we review how to start treatment with Anthony even though he currently denies that his alcohol intake is a problem.

SCREENING FOR ANXIETY DISORDERS

Returning to my consultation with Sallie, I still need to screen for anxiety disorders before deciding on a treatment recommendation.

EXAMPLE 5.4

Screening for anxiety disorders during the consultation

THERAPIST: I have a few more questions to go. Have you ever had a panic attack? [*screening for panic attacks and panic disorder*]

SALLIE: I think so. You mean, those times when a person feels really panicky?

THERAPIST: During a panic attack, a person may definitely feel panicky but may also feel some physical symptoms, such as shortness of breath, chest pain, or dizziness. Have you felt any symptoms like these?

SALLIE: Yes, I did have a panic attack like that about a month ago before an economics test. It was horrible.

THERAPIST: They are horrible. Can you tell me what yours was like?

SALLIE: Well, the professor was passing out the test, and all of a sudden, I felt light-headed and couldn't really breathe. I had no idea what was going on. Then, my hands started to tingle, and I was convinced I was going to pass out. Until I settled down because I realized I actually knew the answers, I felt like I was working through a fog. Honestly though, it was one of the scariest things I have ever experienced. Is this what you are asking about?

THERAPIST: Yes, it is. Panic attacks, by definition, are very scary. Sometimes, during an attack, a person may not know it is a panic attack and might worry that she is dying or going crazy. Did that happen to you?

SALLIE: Umm, yeah. I wasn't going to mention that part because it's sort of embarassing. I thought maybe I had some kind of mini heart attack, but at the student health center they said I was completely fine.

THERAPIST: While panic attacks are unlikely to be due to a medical condition, I'm glad to hear that you already it had it checked out by an internist.

[*screening for agoraphobia*] Sometimes, the panic attack can be so bad that a person might avoid the places that remind her of the attack in order to try to prevent another one. Have you avoided the area where you took the economics test?

SALLIE: No, thank goodness, because most of my tests are in that building!

THERAPIST: [*screening for anxiety symptoms, obsessive–compulsive character traits, and obsessive–compulsive disorder*] Also, in my list of questions: Do you ever notice that you have a thought in your head that really bothers you, so you perform an activity to try to make it go away?

SALLIE: What do you mean?

THERAPIST: Well, some people check things over and over again in their home in order to make sure everything is secure, such as checking to make sure that the door is locked at night or that the stove is turned off.

SALLIE: Oh, I check my front door to make sure it is locked before I go to bed at night.

THERAPIST: How many times do you check it?

SALLIE: Just once.

THERAPIST: Have you ever checked something so many times that you are late to an appointment or has your checking interfered with your daily routine because you are busy making absolutely sure that the object is secure?

SALLIE: Umm, no. I don't think so.

THERAPIST: Have you ever felt compelled to wash or clean anything, including yourself, multiple times to make sure that it is clean?

SALLIE: Well, I am a neat person. I like to make sure that my apartment is clean.

THERAPIST: What I am asking about is a symptom that is beyond basic cleanliness. Have you ever felt convinced that something is dirty and needs recleaning even if you have just finished washing it?

SALLIE: Nope, I am not that obsessive.

THERAPIST: [*screening for posttraumatic stress disorder*] Have you ever had frequent nightmares?

SALLIE: I had a bunch around the time I saw Dr. Anders. I kept dreaming I was locked up in a burning house and couldn't get out. I haven't had one of those dreams for a while, though.

THERAPIST: Have you ever had any flashbacks of traumatic events in your life?

SALLIE: What do you mean . . . flashbacks? Like in the movies when a character remembers the past?

THERAPIST: Yes, that is a good example. When flashbacks happen in real life, the person having them might also reexperience the feelings she had during the original episode.

SALLIE: No, I've never had that.

THERAPIST: Have you ever avoided any place because it reminds you of painful memories?

SALLIE: I don't think so.

THERAPIST: And one more question: Do you startle easily? If a bird flies by you unexpectedly, do you flinch more easily than most other people?

SALLIE: No, I don't do that either. I don't think I really have any of these things.

Example 5.3 screens quickly for common anxiety disorders: panic disorder, agoraphobia, obsessive–compulsive disorder, and posttraumatic stress disorder (PTSD), respectively, based on the symptom criteria presented in the *Diagnostic and Statistical Manual of Mental Disorders*, fourth edition (DSM-IV), the diagnostic manual for psychiatric disorders. Many times, an anxious patient may be bothered by a few of the preceding symptoms without an impairment in daily functioning. In such a case, therapy alone may be sufficient treatment. For more severe symptoms, such as recurrent panic attacks, obsessions or compulsions that interfere with her daily activities for hours at a time, or frightening symptoms consistent with active PTSD (nightmares, flashbacks, avoidance, or an increased startle reflex), a patient deserves psychopharmacological and cognitive-behavioral therapy consultations.

While some clinicians include questions about past physical, emotional, or sexual trauma in the psychological review of systems, others believe that this information is so emotionally charged that the patient should be the first to bring up the topic. One moderate approach would be to ask "Would you feel comfortable telling me about the trauma that caused these symptoms?" for patients reporting a number of PTSD symptoms without a specified cause. Another effective and relatively nonintrusive approach would be to ask about categories of abuse in a questionnaire, as illustrated in our sample at the end of Chapter 4. If the patient is ready and willing to share the details of the trauma, she can document her history in writing. If she is not interested in sharing the information with a relative stranger, it is easier to avoid answering a written question than an oral one.

SCREENING FOR LEARNING DIFFICULTIES

Learning difficulties add persistent stress to everyday life and may increase an individual's risk for an anxiety or mood disorder. For simplicity's sake, we've spared Sallie, but during a review of systems, a clinician can review for signs and symptoms of a profound learning disability.

If a patient describes a persistent history of distractibility, poor grades, and disorganization, she deserves a more thorough neurocognitive evaluation by a clinician knowledgeable in learning disabilities and attention-deficit/hyperactivity disorder. When these diagnoses go unrecognized, they can continue to wreak emotional havoc into adulthood. With the right medication and/or learning support, a patient's performance at school and at work may improve tremendously. Relationships may also benefit as the patient's focus and self-esteem improves.

SCREENING FOR PSYCHOSIS OR BIPOLAR ILLNESS

At this point, I am nearly finished with Sallie's review of systems because her psychiatric history is not very extensive. For patients who seem particularly depressed, withdrawn, hard to talk to, or unusual in a way that is hard to pinpoint, I also screen for psychosis and bipolar illness during the consultation interview. To illustrate how to ask this delicate set of questions, we'll introduce our third fictional patient, Candice Jones. Candice is a depressed, single 45-year-old paralegal who presents with a 2-month history of neurovegetative symptoms so debilitating that she had missed many days of work by the time of our consultation. Before this depression, she had a long history of unstable relationships and some self-injurious behavior during her 20s and 30s. When she is under stress, she has difficulty distinguishing between fantasy and reality. Here is how I would screen for psychosis or mania in her consultation interview.

EXAMPLE 5.5

Screening for psychosis and mania during the consultation interview

I learn about Candice's current depression during the first session. She talks extensively and coherently about all her stressors at work. She

is not currently suicidal. At the beginning of the second session, she seems much worse. She is easily agitated, and has poor eye contact. We start the example after the first 10 minutes of the session.

CANDICE: (*slumping in chair with eyes focused past me and on a painting on the wall behind me*) I don't know what else to say, Dr. Bender. . . . (*Eyes dart around the room*)

THERAPIST: I hear from what you have been telling me that this last month has felt unbearable to you. Sometimes when a person has such a severe depression, as you have, her mind plays tricks on her, but it is too scary to tell anyone because it is so unusual. I don't know if this has happened to you.

CANDICE: (*suspiciously*) What do you mean . . . exactly?

THERAPIST: Well, during a severe depression some people hear voices that only they can hear. Others see things that only they can see. . . .

CANDICE: I do hear voices sometimes. I don't see anything unusual. (*Voice trails off.*)

THERAPIST: What kind of voices do you hear? (*curious, calm tone*)

CANDICE: Well, I hear two actually. These two men yelling at me . . . telling me that I am nothing, that I am useless . . . (*Starts to cry.*)

THERAPIST: It sounds very scary.

CANDICE: It is. (*Crying increases in intensity.*)

THERAPIST: (*Waits quietly. After a minute or so*) Do you want to take a break or may I ask more questions?

CANDICE: (*Wipes her eyes and nose with tissues and takes a few deep breaths.*) It's okay. What else?

THERAPIST: During this very difficult time, have you ever felt that you are receiving any special messages from the TV, radio, or anything else?

CANDICE: No, I don't think so. Well, maybe once. . . . I felt like the newscaster on the 7 o'clock news was mocking me. Is that what you mean?

THERAPIST: Yes, it is. Can you tell me more about what you experienced?

CANDICE: Well, it was last week. I was watching the news, and worried that I might get fired if I don't feel better soon, and then I could see the anchorman looking right at me. When he said, "We'll be right back . . . " I knew he was referring to my voices . . . and then, just as he had predicted, they started screaming at me. (*Looks at me worriedly.*)

THERAPIST: What a day that must have been.

CANDICE: It was one of the worst days of my life.

THERAPIST: Have you ever felt that you have any special powers?

CANDICE: Like ESP? Sometimes I feel I might have a little bit of that.

THERAPIST: Can you tell me more?

CANDICE: Sometimes I think I can tell what people are thinking about me.

THERAPIST: What are they thinking?

CANDICE: Well, they are wondering what's changed about me. I have a very good reputation at the law firm, Dr. Bender. You see, I've worked there for almost 10 years. They must notice that I'm different. I don't even wash my hair anymore.

THERAPIST: Do you ever feel as though they are watching you or following you?

CANDICE: I do think I must be the current subject of most of the office gossip. I just know it.

THERAPIST: What do you think they are saying?

CANDICE: I don't really know, but people seem to be staying away from me at work, or they treat me so gingerly. They know something is up, and something is different.

THERAPIST: Do you ever feel that you could control other people's thoughts or that they could be exerting power over yours?

CANDICE: Not my coworkers, of course, but these two men I hear yelling at me are torturing me. They want me to lose it.

THERAPIST: Does anyone else know about them?

CANDICE: No, of course I haven't told anyone about this. I don't want people to think I am crazy. I know this sounds strange, Dr. Bender, but this is truly happening to me. . . .

THERAPIST: How does it feel to tell me these things?

CANDICE: I'm not sure . . . strange. Maybe . . . maybe a little bit better.

THERAPIST: I can understand why it has been so hard to go to work. In order to recommend the best treatment plan, I also need to know if you have ever experienced what we, as therapists, call mania. In some ways, mania is the opposite of depression. It is an unusual state that lasts more than a few days during which a person doesn't need to sleep, has tons of energy, is able to complete loads of work, and feels incredible, even euphoric.

CANDICE: Well, I felt really happy last year for a few days. I felt wonderful, on top of the world.

THERAPIST: What was happening at that time?

CANDICE: Last May, I met a man named Eric, and in the first weeks of our romance, I felt incredible.

THERAPIST: What was your sleep pattern at that time?

CANDICE: Oh, fine.

THERAPIST: How many hours were you sleeping a night?

CANDICE: Maybe 6 or 7.

THERAPIST: Has there ever been a time in your life when you felt this good, and you had so much energy that, for consecutive days, you only required minimal sleep—maybe just 1–2 hours a night—all without the help of drugs or medications?

CANDICE: Oh, no. I couldn't do that.

When Candice's affect becomes more withdrawn at the beginning of Session 2, I screen for common psychotic symptoms, including, in this order, auditory and visual hallucinations, ideas of reference (receiving special messages), paranoia, thought insertion, and thought broadcasting (the patient experiences that her thoughts are being controlled, or that she can broadcast her thoughts to others, respectively). If Candice's decompensation had emerged during our first session, I wouldn't hesitate to screen for psychosis even earlier in the consultation process.

During this interview, it becomes clear that Candice has auditory hallucinations with hostile content. Her delusion that the TV anchorman was addressing her personally is an example of an idea of reference, a psychotic perspective in which the patient believes general experiences also contain unique meaning intended for her. At first blush, her clinical presentation, including the affectively laden psychotic symptoms, is most consistent with a mood disorder, such as depression with psychotic features. Whatever the final diagnosis, Candice's distress is severe, and she deserves a psychopharmacological consultation as soon as possible.

Candice does not have true paranoia. Her perception of her coworkers is not unreasonable considering the circumstances. Her "special powers" may be intuition about her professional colleagues' reactions to her illness.

Any patient with a severe depression, with or without concurrent psychosis, should be asked about a history of mania. As a psychopharmacologist, I also complete this screening any time I am starting a patient on an antidepressant for the first time. Since antidepressants alone can flip a bipolar patient from depression to mania, they are not recommmended in patients with histories of mania unless they receive a mood stabilizer concurrently.

Candice misunderstands my question about mania when she identifies a very happy time in her life as a manic episode. If she had experienced a true manic episode, the specific symptoms could be delineated, according to DSM-IV criteria, by using the mnemonic DIGFAST (devised by William Falk, MD): D, *d*istractability, I, *i*njudicious behavior and/or *i*mpulsivity, G, *g*randiosity, F, *f*light of ideas, A, increased *a*ctivity, S, *s*leep loss, and T, increased *t*alkativeness. We include further information on the identification and treatment of bipolar illness in the bibliography.

As a beginner, I was worried that my new patients would be offended if I included questions about psychosis in my review of systems. While I do skip the review of systems for psychosis if a patient is high-functioning and without any current risk factors, if I have *any* concern that a patient might have some psychotic symptoms lurking behind her chief complaint, I bite the bullet and ask away. Interestingly enough, the majority of patients, whether or not they are currently psychotic, are relieved that I can talk openly about such frightening symptoms.

As I mentioned at the beginning of this chapter, gathering the developmental history and completing a review of systems has never been my favorite part of this work. However, it is information I need to obtain to make educated treatment recommendations, as I do for Sallie in Chapter 6.

Review of mnemonic for alcohol abuse: CAGE—cut down, annoyed, guilty, eye-opener.

Review of mnemonic for mania: DIGFAST—distractibility, injudicious behavior and/or impulsivity, grandiosity, flight of ideas, increased activity, sleep loss, increased talkativeness

Key words: anxiety disorders, attention-deficit/hyperactivity disorder, auditory processing disorder, bereavement, bipolar disorder, cognitive-behavioral therapy, developmental history, diagnosis, dyslexia, learning disability, mania, mood disorders, obsessive–compulsive disorder (OCD), psychiatric disorders, psychosis, posttraumatic stress disorder (PTSD), rejection, review of systems, substance abuse, symptom history, symptom review, treatment plan

Consultation Summary for the Medical Record

Chief complaint (CC):
Sallie Gane is a 21-year-old single white female college student whose chief
complaint is "My life has been kind of a mess."

Referral source:
The patient's primary care physician at college:
Miranda Newman, MD
617-111-3333

Informant:
The patient: reliable

History of present illness (HPI):
About 6 months prior to her first visit (PTV), the patient was rejected by her boyfriend.
Since then, she has felt "mopey," her appetite has declined, and her ability to concentrate
has decreased. Gradually her symptoms worsened despite her efforts at exercise, socializing, and study.
One week PTV, she had an "all-day" crying spell and decided she needed professional
help.

Past psychiatric history (PPsiH):
During her final months in high school (about 3 years PTV), she purged with and became
dependent upon laxatives. She was hospitalized for 10 days at a psychiatric facility near
her home. Following that, she had a few months of outpatient psychotherapy with Dr. Anders prior to starting college. She reported no other psychiatric treatment.

Substance use:
In addition to laxative abuse, as reported above, she had relatively high alcohol tolerance
during high school. She reports occasional use of marijuana but denies use of any other
recreational substance.

Past medical history (PMH):
Ear infections bilaterally in childhood.
Hand infection at age 10 with one night hospitalization for IV antibiotics.
No head injuries and no loss of consciousness or seizures.

Current medical condition:
A complete physical examination 6 months ago was entirely within normal limits, per pa-
tient report.
Primary care physician at college: Miranda Newman, MD
Primary care physician at home: Rutta Karen, MD

Current medications:
Ibuprofen for menstrual discomfort
Daily multivitamins
Oral contraceptives

Allergies:
Rash associated with penicillin

Family history (FH):
Psychiatric:
Sallie's mother experienced "blues" following her birth.
A maternal uncle had alcohol problems but is now sober.

Medical:
Sallie's brother has suffered from gastrointestional pain and diarrhea.

Social history (SH):
The patient's mother is a real estate agent, and her father manages an electronics store. Her only sibling, Tom, is 6 years younger and is currently in high school.

Mental status examination (MSE):
Sallie Gane is a neatly and casually dressed young woman who appears her stated age and seems to be of roughly normal weight for her height. She is cooperative and engageable throughout the interview, although at times she seems tense and nervous. She has good eye contact. Her speech is normal rate, tone, and volume without any pressure. A review of the neurovegetative symptoms of depression finds that her sleep is normal (7–8 hours nightly), but her interest, motivation, energy, concentration, and appetite are decreased. Her feelings of guilt and self-blame are high; her self-esteem is low. She has no psychomotor agitation or retardation. She occasionally wishes that she would die in an airplane crash, but she has no current suicidal intention, plan, or action. Her thought content is appropriate. She shows no evidence of delusions or hallucinations. Her thought form is well-ordered and logical. Her cognition is grossly intact. Her insight and judgment are fair.

Assessment and plan:
Sallie Gane is a 21-year-old single female college student referred to me by Dr. Newman in primary care for evaluation of Sallie's ongoing symptoms of depression.

Ms. Gane meets the criteria for major depressive disorder, but she has been able to function well in her college studies and does not pose a suicidal threat at this time. Her present concerns revolve around her relationship with her former boyfriend.

At this time, I recommend a trial of psychotherapy to alleviate her distress. If symptoms and functioning worsen, antidepressant medication can be considered. As her psychotherapist, I will remain alert for possible recurrences of her eating disorder or for substance abuse.

Diagnoses:

Axis I:
Major depressive disorder, single episode, mild. (DSM-IV: 296.21)
Eating disorder in remission. (DSM-IV: 307.00)

Axis II:
No diagnosis on Axis II. (DSM-IV: V71.09)

Axis III:
No diagnosis on Axis III.

Axis IV:
Problems related to the patient's social environment.

Axis V:
Global Assessment of Functioning (GAF) Score of 65.

6

Formulating a Treatment Plan

After collecting an adequate history, the therapist needs to formulate a treatment plan that responds to the patient's specific needs. The clinican must decide which type or combination of therapy (psychodynamic therapy, cognitive behavioral therapy, group therapy, or psychopharmaocologic treatment) would be most beneficial for the patient. An overview explaining the process of psychotherapy can reinforce the therapeutic alliance.

In the days of yesteryear, long before the DSMs (*Diagnostic and Statistical Manuals of Mental Disorders*), symptom-based diagnoses, and many different types of therapies, intensive psychoanalytic psychotherapy was often the recommended treatment for patients with psychological suffering. Sometimes it worked wonders. Sometimes it didn't work at all.

Even though I understood that psychoanalytic treatment wasn't for everybody, as a beginner I liked the idea of "one-size-fits-all" treatment. The multiple therapeutic options available to my generation (individual psychodynamic psychotherapy, group psychotherapy, psychopharmacology, and cognitive-behavioral treatment, to name a few) felt intimidating rather than liberating.

It took time and clinical experience to change my limited perspective. As I slowly learned to match each disorder to its most effective treatment, my appreciation for the available wealth of information evolved.

I now try to model myself after my supervisors who stay curious and critical about innovative psychotherapeutic possibilities no matter how long they have been in practice. Dr. Messner is a prime example. He is a trained psychoanalyst, but he is also adept at psychopharmacology and familiar with the basics of cognitive-behavioral and group psychotherapy. He isn't reluctant to refer to these specialized treatments when there is a reason to do so. Similarly, in this book, we will shape each treatment to meet each patient's unique clinical needs.

DECIDING ON A DIAGNOSIS

Before I can recommend a treatment plan for a new patient, I complete a diagnostic formulation using the DSM-IV, the current manual that lists the diagnostic criteria for mental disorders. While overlap can occur, I organize psychiatric disorders into two categories: (1) disorders with targetable symptoms that meet DSM-IV diagnostic criteria (such as mood disorders, thought disorders, anxiety disorders, eating disorders, and substance abuse), and (2) those conditions that are more closely linked to ongoing life stressors (relational problems, occupational problems, adjustment disorders, personality disorders, and the like).

TREATMENT OF DISORDERS
WITH TARGETABLE SYMPTOMS

For the first category of diagnoses, the patient arrives at my office complaining of specific symptoms, such as depressed mood with suicidality and loss of sleep or disabling panic attacks that are disrupting everyday activities. At the very least, psychodynamic psychotherapy can help this group of patients cope with their illnesses and their effect on their work and relationships. Sometimes, with intensive psychotherapy alone, the disabling symptom may also slowly improve.

Understandably, many patients cannot or do not want to wait months (or years) before psychodynamic psychotherapy alone might relieve their debilitating condition. To help the patient return to healthy functioning as soon as possible, I may recommend treatment with medication and/or cognitive-behavioral therapy as well.

A medication evaluation is mandatory in a few instances: (1) when a patient's symptoms of depression and/or anxiety are significantly interfering with her daily functioning, (2) when the patient has a history of mania or psychosis, and (3) when the patient has current manic symptoms, significant agitation, or psychosis.

Cognitive-behavioral therapy (CBT) also focuses on acute symptom alleviation for some anxiety and mood disorders. By identifying underlying irrational beliefs and automatic thoughts, and by teaching cognitive restructuring and behavioral techniques, CBT can provide a skill set that may help alleviate acute emotional distress. For example, a patient who panics in elevators will learn that irrational concern about the physical risk of panic attacks ("If I have another one, I think I might die") may exacerbate baseline nervousness and lead to an avoidance of elevators. After teaching techniques to diminish the power of the irrational belief, the CBT therapist may assign homework so the patient can practice the new skills independently. The therapist might also use behavioral therapy techniques, such as a gradual reexposure to elevators, as part of the treatment plan. As a detailed review of CBT is beyond the scope of this book, our bibliography includes some helpful CBT references.

SPECIALIZED TREATMENT OF SPECIFIC DISORDERS

Patients with eating disorders have targetable symptoms that revolve around diet and exercise, and they often benefit from a multidisciplinary treatment approach. A nutritionist and an internist may be required to assure medical safety. Depending on the specific clinical scenario, the patient may benefit from individual and/or family psychodynamic therapy, medications, and a cognitive-behavioral component. Because these patients are so complicated, I often consult with supervisors experienced with these conditions when I'm unsure how to approach a specific clinical scenario.

As we noted in Chapter 5, the treatment of active substance abusers also requires a unique psychotherapeutic strategy, including a psychopharmacological evaluation. We outline more details of this approach in Chapter 12.

DIAGNOSES THAT PREFERENTIALLY RESPOND TO PSYCHODYNAMIC PSYCHOTHERAPY

Psychodynamic psychotherapy is the preferred treatment if a patient's difficulties revolve around relationships or involve problems of self-esteem. Some of the other common diagnoses that also respond well to psychodynamic psychotherapy include disorders of sexual identity, adjustment disorders, personality disorders, problems related to trauma, abuse or neglect, and maturational crises and associated problems. DSM-IV also lists a number of V codes (conditions that are not considered to be mental illnesses but may be a focus of clinical attention) that often respond to psychotherapy, such as bereavement (V62.82), academic problems (V62.3), occupational problems (V62.2), identity problems (313.82), religious or spiritual problems (V62.89), acculturation problems (V62.4), or phase of life problems (V62.89).

In some cases, group psychotherapy is a useful treatment concurrent with or instead of individual psychotherapy. There are many types of group psychotherapy, including short-term cognitive-behavioral groups that focus on a specific problem (such as panic attacks), theme groups such as those for eating-disordered patients or medically ill patients, and long-term psychodynamic psychotherapy groups that concentrate on interpersonal issues. For patients with recurrent relationship difficulties, a long-term psychodynamic group may be especially useful as the therapy will teach the patient how she is perceived by others. (Please see the bibliography for some recommended texts on group psychotherapy.)

SALLIE'S DIAGNOSIS
AND TREATMENT RECOMMENDATION

Sallie meets the criteria for a mild case of major depressive disorder (DSM-IV: 296.21). She also has an eating disorder, not otherwise specified, in remission (DSM-IV: 307.00). By translating Sallie's difficulties into DSM-IVese, I can summarize her condition in supervision and immediately be understood. If she uses her insurance to pay for treatment, these are the diagnoses that I will note on the claim form. (Please see the consultation summary at the end of Chapter 5 for a concise review of Sallie's assessment.)

After summarizing Sallie's condition with a few numbers, we feel the need to add a disclaimer. While a diagnosis is a necessary part of her treatment, it doesn't even start to capture the complexity of her situation. DSM-IV is always a simplification. The truth is that every patient is a complex human being with unique strengths, traits, and yearnings.

I will recommend to Sallie that she start weekly individual psychotherapy because she is intensely distressed, is grieving a loss, and has a history of interpersonal problems. Based on the information I've gathered during the consultation, Sallie's problems are best served by a more traditional psychodynamic treatment, rather than by a symptom-based intervention such as cognitive-behavioral therapy. While she is in crisis, we also think she would benefit most from the one-on-one attention of individual psychotherapy. Over time, if individual psychotherapy does not provide enough emotional support, or if Sallie wishes to understand more how she interacts with others in a therapeutic environment, I might consider an additional referral to a long-term psychotherapy group that focuses on relationship issues.

Currently, I'm not recommending cognitive-behavioral treatment or medication. If Sallie started to have panic attacks (or some other targetable symptom) within the context of her many stressors, I would reconsider adjunctive CBT with a therapist specially trained in this modality. Medication isn't currently indicated because Sallie's daily functioning is not severely impaired, and she is not at risk for suicide.

As I make my treatment recommendation, I explain the process of therapy to Sallie.

EXAMPLE 6.1

Explaining the process of psychotherapy to a new patient

THERAPIST: How has it felt talking to me over these last few meetings?

SALLIE: It has been okay, I guess.

THERAPIST: As I think about what we have talked about, I believe psychotherapy will be able to help you. I think the distress that you are feeling about Charlie would improve through talking to me weekly about your concerns.

SALLIE: You really think so?

THERAPIST: Yes, but there are also alternatives: cognitive-behavioral treatment, group therapy, and medications, to name a few. You could even consider no treatment at all. I'll be glad to explain the other treatments if you wish.

SALLIE: But you think psychotherapy would be the best type of treatment for me?

THERAPIST: Yes, as I see it, if you could have figured out this situation with Charlie intellectually, you would have by now. I think the way for you to feel better is to learn more about your inner experience, learning with your heart, not only with your head. Psychotherapy can help you do this.

SALLIE: You're right that it has been a problem of the heart. I feel like my heart was broken. But I don't really understand what I have to do to feel better.

THERAPIST: Psychotherapy will allow you to get closer to inner feelings by using a format similar to what we have been using, but with some differences. First, I think it would be good to continue to meet once a week for 50 minutes, but I won't be directing the meeting with a list of questions as I have done during the consultation, and I won't be taking as many notes. Instead, I'll want to hear about your current concerns. When I think it will help, I'll try to add my observations and will probably ask an occasional question. Your task will be to talk about whatever is on your mind, trying not to edit. [*I introduce the concept of free association.*]

SALLIE: Yeah, but what good is that going to do?

THERAPIST: It can be helpful to confide in someone in detail about your experience with Charlie. You may also start to feel better as you gain some perspective and learn from what happened.

SALLIE: But, I talk to my friend, Gwen, about Charlie all the time. No offense, Dr. Bender, but I don't really understand how this is supposed to be different.

THERAPIST: No offense taken. I'm glad you feel comfortable asking these questions.

A psychotherapist can provide more objectivity than a friend as well as specific knowledge and training for healing the wounds of difficult life events like yours. When Gwen hears about the situation with Charlie, she might relate it to her own dating experiences, and her input will be influenced by her personal relationship with you. As a therapist, I can be more objective, and my training has centered on helping people with relationship difficulties.

SALLIE: Yeah, but all that training won't bring Charlie back!

THERAPIST: Well, that's true, but it might help you to discover ways to calm and to soothe your feelings and to prevent a tormenting breakup like this from happening again.

SALLIE: Oh. . . .

THERAPIST: During our work together, you might have feelings about things I say, including a feeling that I may not have understood something. If this happens, I hope that you will tell me.

SALLIE: How will that help?

THERAPIST: Together we can learn a lot if we are open to talking about our relationship. Psychotherapy is a process that deals with three sets of relationships: present, past, and the one between you and me. By sharing with me any feelings you have about our relationship, we might learn more about the other relationships in your life. Any feelings about what goes on in this room can be an important part of our work together. [*This is an adapted explanation of transference.*]

SALLIE: I can try, but I am pretty shy about being direct about things like that.

THERAPIST: That's natural. I'll try to help. This is why I am telling you now that I welcome more openness. Other paths to learn about one's inner life are through mental images, daydreams, and night dreams. If any occur to you, feel free to bring them in.

SALLIE: You have got to be kidding! This is starting to feel a little like psychobabble.

THERAPIST: (*calmly, and not defensively*) Dreams and other forms of imagination can sometimes be very helpful in learning about inner parts of life that are difficult to think about otherwise. The ideas and feelings they bring up can be useful in psychotherapy. I just wanted you to know they are welcome here.

SALLIE: So, how long does this take? When will I feel better?

THERAPIST: It's difficult to predict. One of our goals is to enable you to feel better as soon as possible. How are you feeling now compared to when we first met?

SALLIE: About the same. It's just hard being patient. I want to feel better immediately.

THERAPIST: I can understand that. Usually, it takes a little time to feel better, and it is hard to be patient.

In about 10 minutes or less, and without using any psychological jargon, I've taught Sallie Gane about free association, transference, and the usefulness of dreams in psychotherapy. Because I described the difference between the consultation process and ongoing psychotherapy, the apparent lack of structure in the sessions that follow will be viewed, appropriately, as deliberate, with a specific purpose. My change in style from the last session of the consultation to the first session of the psychotherapy will now be understood and expected.

Sallie also requests immediate relief, a common request from a new patient in crisis. Although I can't promise rapid improvement, cognitive or behavioral interventions that maximize coping skills can be integrated within the psychodynamic treatment to provide a measure of early relief. Some examples of these techniques are outlined in Chapter 9, which focuses on crisis intervention. There is also great comforting power in feeling understood. Often, with an empathic therapist who listens carefully, the patient will start to feel a little better after the first few meetings.

IF YOU DON'T WANT TO TREAT THE PATIENT AFTER YOU HAVE COMPLETED THE CONSULTATION

As a trainee, my supervisors recommended that I work with numerous patients with a range of psychiatric disorders in order to gain experience. With this advice in mind, I sometimes hesitated to continue treating a patient after the consultation was completed. For instance, I might want to hold my open session slot for a male psychotherapy patient if my entire caseload were female.

Early on, I also referred some patients who were too frightening to other providers. During my first year as a therapist, I refused to treat any actively suicidal outpatient because I was scared that my inexperience would be fatal. Experience has helped me feel more and more comfortable treating a wide range of patients, but in the beginning, I was more fearful.

Rarely, the reason I didn't want to treat a patient was much more personal and much more embarrassing. What if I had an aversion to talking to Sallie and felt little empathy for her troubles? What if she reminded me of a bully from grade school or a snotty girl from junior high dance class? My first stop would be supervision to try to understand and to work through my difficulty. But sometimes, even with the best of intentions, I wasn't able to shake the "emotional block." (For more discussion of how a therapist's reaction to a patient can affect the treatment, please see Chapter 16 on transference and countertransference.)

If I had persistent or profound trouble connecting with a patient from the get-go, it wasn't in anyone's best interest for me to continue as the therapist after the consultation was completed. I would try to learn from the experience, but I would need to trust my instincts. If I didn't feel able to treat the patient, I'd refer the person to a clinician who could be an eager and engaged collaborator.

Unfortunately, while it is often easy for a therapist to refer a patient to another clinician, it can be very upsetting to be on the receiving end of a transfer. As a guilt-ridden beginning therapist, it's easy to complicate the already loaded situation by minimizing or denying the patient's hurt feelings to alleviate one's own distress ("I know you expected to work with me, but I think you'll like Dr. Smith even better anyway") or by delaying the news until the consultation's final session.

In general, patients are rarely delighted to learn that they will be passed off to another clinician after the consultation is completed. They digest the information more easily if they learn about the transfer during the first or second consultation meeting and have time to process their disappointment.

EXAMPLE 6.2

The therapist sensitively refers the new patient to another clinician early in the consultation

At the Beginning of the Second Session

THERAPIST: Before we start the second session today, I wanted to know if you had any thoughts about our last session.

SALLIE: No, not really.

THERAPIST: I learned enough in our first session to recognize that I don't feel qualified to be your therapist but can complete the consultation if you are willing. At the end of the consultation, when we decide on a treatment plan, I'll be able to refer you to a clinician I know who would be most appropriate to take over your treatment.

SALLIE: Why can't you see me?

THERAPIST: It is a matter of professional judgment about what's best for you. [*I am deliberately vague to avoid an in-depth discussion about this issue.*]

SALLIE: Oh, I was hoping I could continue with you.

THERAPIST: I appreciate your saying that. How do you feel hearing this news?

SALLIE: Crappy, and bummed. I must be hitting a new low to be rejected by a therapist!

THERAPIST: In view of your experience with Charlie, I can understand how this can feel like a rejection to you. It is hard to complete a consultation and then switch treaters, but with the information we review together in the next few meetings, I will be able to match you up with one of my colleagues.

SALLIE: Someone you know?

THERAPIST: Yes, I will try to refer you to someone whose work I know well.

As I've gained experience as a psychiatrist, referrals to other therapists have become a relatively easy process. I refer to my professional network. During 6 years of post–medical school training, I've logged hundreds of hours of supervision with very experienced clinicians and with peer supervision groups. If I cannot take on a new patient, I refer with confidence to my colleagues, because I know their work well and trust their abilities.

NOTE TAKING

I always regret when I don't tell new patients that I usually don't take notes in the sessions that follow the consultation. When I'm writing, the patient may feel her story is noteworthy (excuse the pun). When I don't explain my abrupt decrease in note taking, she may easily misinterpret the change as a reduction in my attention and a waning of interest.

Some therapists have an uncanny ability to listen, to maintain eye contact, and to jot legible words simultaneously, and they may continue to take notes as a therapy progresses. Even if you are one of these talented few, this procedure also travels with its own potential difficulties. A former patient of mine, whom I'll call Anne, once described how she scrutinized her previous therapist's note taking. She watched her therapist's hands carefully, noticing when she picked up her pen or put it down. Over time, Anne began to feel upset when the therapist didn't take notes after she had related an especially sensitive story. A simple action had become replete with emotional meaning. It was unfortunate that Anne never shared her feelings about this issue with her therapist. The therapy would have benefitted from an open discussion of her concerns.

PROCESS NOTES

Before I begin to work with Sallie in an ongoing therapy (because I've created her to be a patient I am interested in and able to work with), let's touch base about process notes.

My future therapy sessions with Sallie won't have a predictable pattern. The content of each session will depend on Sallie's current concerns. After each therapy hour is completed, I'll write some "process notes" that will allow me to re-create the therapeutic process for my supervisor or for my own future reference.

During my first months of training, it took a full hour to record the content from a 50-minute session. Luckily, with more practice, the process of writing process notes became more expeditious. Now I don't try to record the session verbatim, but only note the key moments of the session, so I'll remember them later on. I complete my process notes in the 10 minutes between patients when my recall for a session's material is most vivid.

To organize the notes, I divide a plain sheet of paper in half with a vertical line (or fold) down the center. On the left side of the paper, I write down as much as I can remember of the session's most meaningful moments (including names of important people in the patient's life so I'll have them for future reference). Then, on the right side of the paper, I write any questions, ideas, or feelings I may have had during the hour. During supervision, I'll use my notes to formulate my questions and guide the discussion.

EXAMPLE 6.3

An excerpt from a session followed by a typical process note that abbreviates the action and formulates the therapist's questions

Sallie rushes in 15 minutes late.

SALLIE: I am so, so sorry. Traffic was terrible. I don't know why it is so hard to get here. My new job makes it hard to get here on time. Did I tell you? I got a work-study position at the library. I am REALLY sorry. I just can't leave early to make it on time.

THERAPIST: It was difficult to leave enough time to get here?

SALLIE: Yes. My new boss is difficult, and I want to make a good impression. Maybe I could have made it if I had left the library 10 minutes earlier, but I didn't want to ask for any special favors. Not during my first week anyway.

THERAPIST: So leaving 10 minutes early one afternoon a week doesn't feel right?

SALLIE: It might be okay once I get settled in the job. My new boss is tough, but she also seems fair. She said that she would be flexible with our schedules because she knows that we have other commitments. I just don't want to push it.

THERAPIST: It feels difficult to ask for the favor. Can you tell me why?

SALLIE: I just don't want to jeopardize anything.

THERAPIST: I can understand why you might be careful asking for favors during your first week on the job, but it also sounds like your relationship with her feels somewhat fragile—that one minor wrong step might jeopardize your position at work?

SALLIE: Yes, that's it.

THERAPIST: Can you tell me more about how that feels?

SALLIE: I don't know. I just get so scared. People can like you one minute and ignore you the next for no apparent reason.

THERAPIST: Have you had other experiences in which people liked you 1 minute but ignored you the next?

SALLIE: Well, didn't that happen with Charlie? It seemed to be going great from my point of view, but then we broke up and I still don't totally get it.

THERAPIST: The breakup with Charlie was so upsetting because you had invested so much in the relationship, and it was unclear, at least at first, why it didn't work out.

SALLIE: I still don't get it. Do you?

THERAPIST: I don't, but I think we will learn more as we continue to work together. Had you ever experienced such an unanticipated change in a relationship before Charlie?

SALLIE: I guess it has happened before, but usually with girlfriends. Amanda, my best friend in elementary school, moved away when I was in 9th grade. Even though we promised to write every day, we stopped almost immediately. I felt so upset because she was my number one best friend, and then she basically disappeared from my life after she moved.

In 10th grade, I became very good friends with a girl named Dawn, and the same sort of thing happened when we went to different colleges. This time it didn't hurt as much because I sort of expected it. But I still don't get it. Other people manage to keep their friends even if they switch schools. (*Sniffles, and looks very upset.*)

THERAPIST: Some of the important female relationships in your life have not worked out the way you hoped.

SALLIE: That's true, I guess.

THERAPIST: It would make sense that you might also have some concerns about our relationship, and whether I will be stable or leave you as the others have.

SALLIE: I don't know. It's scary to talk about it.

THERAPIST: It might feel scary the first time we talk openly about our relationship, but I hope over time that we can learn more about it together.

PROCESS NOTE FOR SALLIE GANE, JANUARY 2

SALLIE: Sorry. Traffic. work study position. *15 minutes late.* Couldn't leave early

SB [*my initials*]: Difficult to get here?	*(Is there any other reason she can't get here on time? When should I bring this up?)*
SALLIE: Can't ask boss to leave early.	*I feel nervous. Will Sallie quit treatment?*

SB: So even leaving 10 minutes early once a week feels wrong?

Ask supervisor what she/he would have said here. My comment didn't seem like the best choice.

SALLIE: Don't want to jeopardize the relationship.

Does Sallie worry that if she takes one misstep, that our relationship would also suffer? When should I bring this up directly?

SB: Relationships are fragile?

SALLIE: Can't depend on good relationships.

SB: Ever happened before?

SALLIE: Charlie.

SB: Ever happened before?

Did I move off of Charlie too quickly?

SALLIE: Friend Sarah—up til 9th grade—lost touch; Dawn—high school, same story.

Sallie looked very upset. Should I push for more information? What would be the right thing to say here?

SB: Female relationships don't work out as you would hope.

Should I have asked more about her mom instead? Is it too early and/or too intense to talk about the therapeutic relationship so directly? Asked about her relationship with me.

SALLIE: Too scary to talk about it.

I finish my training in 3 years. Already I feel guilty about leaving Sallie.

My prowess as a psychotherapist improved dramatically when I started taking process notes on a regular basis for my own benefit and for supervision. I still write process notes for each session with every patient. In intermittent supervision, the reconstructions of the sessions help my supervisors critique my work constructively, and the overview often inspires a deeper understanding of the patient's struggles.

Process notes also helped me identify the clinical situations I was most nervous about as a beginning psychotherapist. What should I do if a patient is late? How do I talk to a patient about vacations? A list of complicated, interesting, and anxiety-provoking clinical scenarios emerged. We developed the next several chapters in response to this list. By focusing on common clinical predicaments and providing some strategies for the clinician, they might provide a useful review even for experienced therapists.

Key words: adjustment disorder, anxiety disorders, bereavement, bipolar disorder, cognitive-behavioral therapy, developmental history, diagnosis, DSM-IV, grief, group psychotherapy, interpersonal problems, loss, personality traits, process notes, psychiatric disorders, psychopharmacology, psychosis, rejection, substance abuse, symptom history, symptom review, treatment plan

Part II
Frame and Variations

7

The Frame

Psychotherapy can seethe with emotional intensity. Therapists follow practice guidelines collectively known as "the frame" to create a safe environment that maintains the therapist's relative objectivity and contains the patient's emotional overflows. While at first the novice patient and therapist may find these standards of practice random and unnecessary, they are indispensable because they protect the integrity of the therapeutic relationship. Limits around scheduling, the beginning and ending of sessions, personal self-disclosures by the therapist, and outside contacts need to be explained clearly and sensitively.

The "frame" refers to a set of behavioral guidelines that define the patient's and the therapist's roles within the confidential therapeutic environment. The term "the frame" is shorthand for "the frame of reference" that defines the differences between a psychotherapeutic relationship and a personal relationship.

From the first meeting, features of "the frame" pervade a psychotherapy. A stable meeting time is established as soon as possible. The session begins and ends at predetermined times. Fees are negotiated as necessary. Any changes in these arrangements that affect the treatment, such as a vacation, are discussed ahead of time. The therapist divulges relatively little personal information about herself, and the patient and the therapist do not interact socially. With a few exceptions defined by law, information about the treatment is never divulged to anyone without express permission unless the patient's safety or the safety of another individual is at risk.

Some rules provided by the frame make obvious sense. It's clear to most why a romantic relationship between a patient and her therapist is unethical and emotionally harmful. Other guidelines may seem more obscure, and many beginning therapists harbor some covert questions about these aspects of the frame. For instance, while many new therapists secretly wonder why a therapist and a patient can't be friends, many trainees are too embarassed to ask a teacher why this rule exists.

Let's consider the possible ramifications of a social relationship between a therapist and her patient. I'll make myself the fall guy with a new hypothetical patient we'll call Zoe. To complicate matters, let's make Zoe a reasonably stable person. She starts psychotherapy seeking help with career issues. She is also an avid tennis player. In our virtual scenario, I'm a tennis player also, and both Zoe and I are in need of a tennis partner. This information "slips" out during a therapy session, and Zoe asks me if I would like to play tennis with her this weekend. Against my better judgment, I agree. How will the psychotherapy be affected?

From the moment I play tennis with Zoe, our relationship's dynamic is irrevocably altered. As a friendship naturally moves toward the social norm of give and take, it cannot coexist with the previous one-sided therapeutic relationship that focused primarily on Zoe.

To play devil's advocate, it's always possible that our tennis game will be the beginning of a great unambivalent, uncomplicated friendship that lasts a lifetime. Meanwhile, Zoe will have to find a new therapist, but it's worth it because our friendship is so lasting and enriching.

Actually, this lovely outcome is about as likely as winning a lottery. A relationship born out of a betrayal (in this case, my betrayal of my professional role) will rarely flourish. As patient and therapist, Zoe and I had agreed on a set of goals for her treatment. Losing me as a therapist but gaining me as a friend may seem like a plum opportunity from afar, but, by losing me as an objective listener, Zoe has just sustained an emotional loss.

I also shouldn't assume that Zoe doesn't really need or want therapy. While "career concerns" may seem like a vanilla topic, discussions in therapy about her dreams for her future may be complicated by a host of complex emotions—emotions she might confide in a therapist but never tell a new friend.

Zoe may also be using "career concerns" as a ticket to enter treatment and to talk about a number of relationship difficulties that are troubling her. What if my friendship with Zoe runs into the same complicated problems that she has experienced in other close relationships? Once again, Zoe gets hurt, but since I'm involved, I'm no longer available as an objective listener. Due to an understandable mistrust of the profession, she may avoid seeking out future therapists to process her experience with me.

It would be very different if Zoe ever felt rejected by me within the confines of our professional relationship. Within a therapeutic relationship, I can be relatively objective. We could talk about her experience and attain a deeper emotional understanding of the process. (For more about this sort of event, please see Chapter 15.) But, as a tennis partner, I've lost my unique perspective and my credibility in relation to Zoe. She doesn't get help with her relationship problems, and the friendship fails—not a good treatment outcome.

Many patients are tempted to draw their therapist into personal relationships to satisfy unfulfilled needs in their own lives. If the therapist tries to fulfill the patient's wishes rather than to help the patient understand her yearnings for closeness, her good intentions lead her onto a slippery slope. Any decrease in boundaries tends to accelerate once it starts, to the detriment of all involved. Ultimately, my role as a therapist is not to become the friend or partner that is missing but to help the patient develop the internal capacity to enrich her own life.

The structure of the therapeutic relationship enables the therapist to maintain adequate objectivity. The patient also benefits by the predictable beginning and end of each meeting. The clearly defined session exit may help the patient to bear the expression of painful and upsetting feelings. The scheduled future session can pick up any matters not fully settled.

MINOR FRAME ALTERATIONS WITHIN A THERAPY

If both the therapist and the patient know the specific rules that define the psychotherapeutic relationship, it is meaningful when the patient (or therapist!) bends or breaks the frame. For instance, the frame is affected when a patient is repeatedly 10–15 minutes late to her session. Even if she repeatedly blames traffic for her tardiness, I'd wonder (silently at first and then aloud) what prevents her from attending a session in its entirety.

If psychotherapy didn't follow clearly outlined starting and stopping times, I might never notice that a patient repeatedly misses the first third of her session. It wouldn't be reasonable or even fair to wonder whether the recurrent tardiness was some kind of emotional indicator. On the other hand, if both my patient and I know that the session starts and ends at predetermined times, it *is* meaningful if she repeatedly misses a significant chunk of our time together. In psychotherapy, we often discover that recurrent events, such as these repeated late arrivals, are rarely random. Over time, the patient and I may learn that there is an underlying, maybe unconscious, reason for the pattern of tardiness. (In Chapter 10 we will discuss how to address a patient's recurrent late arrivals.)

In therapy, every attempt needs to be made to translate action into spoken feelings and thoughts. If a patient is recurrently late, eventually I'll try to discuss this with her in a noncritical and open manner. If a patient wants to change the parameters of our meetings by having a 30- or 90- minute session or by seeing me twice a week, we will talk about the issue thoughtfully and deliberately before doing anything that changes our initial therapeutic contract. Talking after a change has been actualized isn't nearly as effective. Once a treatment's structure is modified to suit my patient's desires, she might lack sufficient internal motivation to delve into the emotional meaning behind her request.

Beginning therapists may be tempted to alter the frame in subtle ways as "errors of kindness," but frame violations may increase the risk of a poor treatment outcome. For instance, a beginning therapist may be tempted to shield a needy patient from treatment fees by "forgetting" to fill out the appropriate clinic paperwork. While this action may seem altruistic, ultimately, this type of frame violation might impair the therapeutic process. When the patient realizes that she isn't being billed, she may feel thrilled at first, but feelings of obligation toward the therapist, doubts about the therapist's honesty and loyalty to her clinic or institution, and even concerns about the therapist's passive–aggressive behavior may follow. A seemingly benevolent procedure can become countertherapeutic.

This section of the book will illustrate how a therapist can use alterations in the frame as opportunities for exploration and discussion. The topics covered reflect the ones that gave me the most anxiety: how to set the fee and to bill, handle telephone calls and crises, respond to patients who arrive late, and manage confidentiality. Since most people don't talk about these issues outside of psychotherapy, it is easy for a novice therapist to become wordless when faced with a frame issue that requires frank discussion. We hope to provide you with some guidance that can help you broach these topics with your patients. Then an open, thoughtful, and therapeutically beneficial dialogue can follow.

> **Key words:** appointments, boundaries, contract violations, fiduciary duty, fees, frame, frequency of sessions, intensive psychotherapy, interview structure, objectivity, patient's questions, perspective, termination of interview, therapeutic alliance, therapeutic contract, therapeutic frame, therapeutic relationship

8

Setting the Fee and Billing

The exchange of money for services is an intrinsic part of every psychotherapy. At first, many altruistic therapists are uncomfortable accepting money for their services. Even some experienced therapists may have difficulty talking to patients directly about money.

We provide some guidelines to help you to set a fee and to bill patients, whether they are paying out-of-pocket, their insurance company is footing the bill, or their care is subsidized by a clinic. The therapist's goal is to provide a clear expectation regarding payment and then to talk sensitively with the patient about her reactions to the guidelines.

As a novice therapist, talking to patients about money was more uncomfortable for me than talking to them about sex. While I felt a little nervous the first time I listened to a patient's intimate sexual concerns, I considered it a privilege when a patient could trust me enough to share such sensitive information. In contrast, discussions about fees and payment felt self-serving in a treatment that deals in the currency of empathy and emotions. Monetary discussions in a psychotherapy are unique because the focus is on the therapist's agenda rather than the patient's needs.

As a novice, I wished there was a way I could practice therapy without having to discuss payment with my patients. A generation ago, my wish would have been fulfilled—at least sometimes. Generous insurance companies often provided years of psychotherapy reimbursement without requiring the disclosure of confidential patient information. With today's health care management, these types of insurance plans are practically nonexistent. Instead, basic mental health insurance coverage generally provides a limited number of psychotherapy sessions. For any additional treatment, the patient and the therapist independently negotiate a fee and payment method.

During my first 2 years as a trainee, I treated only clinic patients, and the MGH department of financial services took care of most monetary issues, including the setting of the fee and collecting payment.

In Massachusetts, as in many other places, every hospital provides a certain percentage of completely free health care, including psychotherapy. As a trainee, these recipients comprised the most desirable patients. I didn't have to report confidential information about these patients to an insurance company. The therapy was completely subsidized as long as the patient's financial situation didn't improve substantially. Patients received therapy, I received my paycheck for working with clinic patients, and money was never an issue. What could be better?

Then a few unexpected treatment issues emerged. Some of my free-care patients had a difficult time taking advantage of the therapy when they felt constantly guilty about getting something for nothing. Others would treat the free service as expendable by forgetting to show or arriving late for scheduled appointments. When I finished my adult psychiatry residency and offered to continue privately with some of these patients for a very reduced fee, many of them declined. Despite the fact that they were satisfied with my care, they chose to receive therapy for no charge with a new clinic provider than to pay for treatment with me.

Slowly, I began to understand the clinical advantages of paying for psychotherapy. As my experience with the free-care patients demonstrated, it's easy to devalue a process that is free. In addition, the fee is a useful tool that defines the limitations and possibilities of the therapeutic relationship. While the collaboration between a therapist and a patient is one of mutual regard and respect, with the focus exclusively on a patient's private emotional concerns, it is still a fee-for-service enterprise. The payment defines the relationship as a working entity, rather than as a substitute for other sustaining relationships.

SETTING THE FEE

During my residency, I could wax poetic on money's necessary role in psychotherapy, but the clinic continued to manage all monetary issues for my patients. When I started a small private practice before graduation, I felt uncomfortable talking to patients directly about fees and payment for therapy. My motivation to master this topic intensified overnight.

Early on, I'm sure that my patients could sense my ambivalence about charging for my services. A new patient would rarely ask details about my fee early in the treatment, so it was very easy for me to make mistakes of omission and delay a discussion about monetary issues until later in treatment.

EXAMPLE 8.1

The therapist does not review her fee with the private practice patient early in treatment and then ends up accepting a much lower fee

During my comprehensive consultation with Sallie Gane, I "forget" to discuss my fee and she does not ask about it. We decide to continue working together after the consultation is completed. At the month's end, I hand her a bill for my services.

THERAPIST: This covers our work together during September. Here is how my billing works. I will give you a bill at the beginning of each month and expect payment by the end of the month. [*I hand Sallie a bill for four sessions totaling $400.00.*]

SALLIE: Oh . . . okay. (*Looks at the bill.*) $400.00!

THERAPIST: You were expecting a different amount?

SALLIE: Ummm, well . . . yes! You didn't tell me you were $100.00 an hour!

THERAPIST: Well, I thought you were aware that this is the average fee in this area. Didn't your primary care doctor tell you this when she referred you to me?

SALLIE: No, I thought my insurance would pay for this. Can I give this bill to my insurance? Are you an EntropyMedical provider?

THERAPIST: Actually, I am not part of that insurance plan. [*I feel guilty and uncomfortable.*] Let's think together how we can approach this in a way that will feel fair to you.

SALLIE: Well, I think I could afford $200.00 a month. . . .

THERAPIST: Okay, that's fine.

In Example 8.1, I feel so uncomfortable and guilty about charging for my services that I don't discuss monetary issues during the first sessions, and then immediately agree to a 50% reduction of payment when Sallie balks at her bill. I'm not independently wealthy, so by agreeing to accept a reduced fee, I'll have to work an extra hour every other week to make up the lost income.

Sallie didn't broach the subject of my fee during our first four meetings. When I didn't mention the cost of the treatment, she may have had a surreptitious wish that the therapy might be free. My reluctance to talk openly about my fee is countertherapeutic because it colludes with her regressive fantasy.

It's best to talk openly about fees and payment very early in the treatment. Often, I'll ask the patient during the first phone call if she would like to discuss my fee on the phone or wait until the first visit. I might also inquire whether she intends to use her health insurance to pay for treatment. This procedure prevents any future misunderstanding or disappointment if the patient expects to use her insurance to subsidize her treatment, only to discover that I am not a provider on this insurance plan during the first visit.

Whether on the phone or in my office, the first conversation about fees can follow a somewhat standardized format.

EXAMPLE 8.2

The therapist discusses her fee and insurance issues during the first phone call

Midway through My First Phone Call with Sallie

THERAPIST: Do you have health insurance?

SALLIE: I have EntropyMedical insurance through school. I think it pays for therapy.

THERAPIST: Unfortunately, I am not an EntropyMedical provider, so the insurance will not be able to offset my fee if you want to work with me.

SALLIE: My primary doctor thought you would be a good therapist for me. Is there any way to work it out?

THERAPIST: My fee per session is $100.00 if you are willing to pay out of pocket.

SALLIE: Oh, gosh I didn't expect that much.

THERAPIST: What were you expecting?

SALLIE: I don't know. I thought you wouldn't charge so much since you see students. I guess I thought it might cost $35.00 an hour or something like that. I think $100.00 is too expensive for me. Umm, what should I do now?

THERAPIST: We have a number of options. If you can obtain a list of

EntropyMedical providers from your insurance company, I would be happy to review the list with you on the phone. If I know any of the therapists, I can help you choose one from the list. I can also refer you to a clinician who might be able to slide his payment scale, although it still may not be as low as you might like. Also, I have the numbers of a few community clinics in your area that could provide therapy at a lower rate. What sounds good to you?

SALLIE: I don't know.

THERAPIST: [*I wait patiently in silence. I sense Sallie's unspoken wish that I make a special exception to treat her at a below market rate, but I do not make this a treatment option.*]

SALLIE: I guess maybe I could ask my parents to help me out so I could at least see you for a few visits, and then see if I want to continue.

THERAPIST: Sure, that is another option.

SALLIE: What do we do next?

THERAPIST: Well, we've set a meeting time for 4:00 P.M. this Wednesday. Would you like to keep this time and discuss my fee with your parents before our meeting?

SALLIE: Oh, that's good, I think. That will give me some time to work on this.

THERAPIST: If it doesn't look like you will be able to pay my fee, please call me at least 48 hours in advance of our appointment to review some of the other options I mentioned. What's most important is that you get some help with the problems you are struggling with.

SALLIE: Okay. Thanks.

If a new patient prefers to discuss monetary issues during her first session, I bring up the topic midway through the meeting. I also try to finish any discussion about fees and administrative details with 10 minutes to spare so we can return briefly to the important clinical issues and plan for further meetings.

The scenario becomes a bit more complicated if I am a provider under the patient's insurance plan. (We will refer to EntropyMedical as our prototypical managed care insurance plan.) Unlike the insurance plans of the past, many current health plans require psychotherapists to divulge patients' personal information before they will provide coverage for more than a few sessions each year. While the complex issues of managed health care may sometimes feel overwhelming, I try to discuss them openly with my patients so they can make an informed decision about their treatment.

EXAMPLE 8.3

Discussing managed care as payment for psychotherapy and
how to set a reduced fee

SALLIE: I have EntropyMedical insurance through school. Can I use it to
see you?

THERAPIST: I think you should be able to. I am an EntropyMedical provider. Are you familiar with how the insurance works?

SALLIE: Not really.

THERAPIST: The insurance provides full payment for eight sessions each
year. Then, if we see that it might be useful to continue treatment,
I'll talk to an insurance coordinator and give her an update on our
work together. The insurance company will decide whether it will
pay for additional sessions.

SALLIE: Do you tell them a lot about me? I don't feel comfortable with
them knowing my business.

THERAPIST: It is important for you to know that while the insurance
company will try to set up a confidential situation between the coordinator and myself, some or all of the information will be entered
into EntropyMedical's computer system.

   The information isn't quite as protected as if we were working
without the input of the company. The benefit, of course, is that
your treatment will be supported by your insurance.

   When I talk to insurance providers, I try to be as general as
possible, but sometimes they won't authorize further visits without
specific information.

SALLIE: Does the information stay private?

THERAPIST: Most insurance companies try to maintain confidentiality,
but I don't know who will have access to your information. For
your particular situation with EntropyMedical, you may want to
call to learn details of their protocol.

SALLIE: What if I don't want you to talk to anyone?

THERAPIST: In that case, you have your first eight sessions covered, and I
will only need to provide them with a diagnosis.

SALLIE: What's my diagnosis?

THERAPIST: It's difficult to say after only one session, but it may be adjustment disorder with depressed mood, or major depression. Both
diagnoses reflect the distress you have suffered after your breakup
with Charlie.

SALLIE: This is so complicated!

THERAPIST: I agree that it can feel overwhelming, especially the first time you learn about a managed care system like this.

SALLIE: What happens after the eight sessions if I don't want to use my insurance any more?

THERAPIST: At that point, I will charge you my regular fee per session, which is $100.00.

SALLIE: Since I'm a student, is there any way that you could reduce your fee for me?

THERAPIST: What portion of $100.00 would you be able to pay?

SALLIE: Umm. Maybe $70.00?

THERAPIST: What is that based on?

SALLIE: I could earn $70.00 a week working extra hours at the library or tutoring.

THERAPIST: Seventy dollars a session is a bit low, but I would agree to a reduced fee of $80 a session.

SALLIE: I'm not sure, but I think I could probably manage that. I think I'll want to keep working after my eight sessions are up. I doubt that I'll totally understand what happened with Charlie after only 2 months of meetings.

THERAPIST: I think you're right that it often takes time to truly understand an emotional event like the breakup with Charlie. We'll consider $80 your fee for now, and if your financial situation changes, we can reconsider the fee at that time.

You should also know how I do my billing. Unless you would prefer to pay me at each visit, I'll give you a bill at the beginning of each month; you'll have until the end of the month to pay me.

SALLIE: Oh, okay. Thank you so much for reducing the fee. That really helps, and I am glad that I can continue to see you.

THERAPIST: I am glad that we were able to work something out as well.

Before discussing out-of-pocket treatment, I try to converse openly with the patient about managed care's simultaneous support of and interference with psychotherapy. Due to financial limitations, not all patients have the choice to pay for treatment out of pocket. Moreover, early in treatment, a patient may not care about issues of confidentiality and may feel understandably entitled to her health care benefits. The treater's responsibility is to explain the issues involved, especially the implications of waiving confidentiality, so the patient can weigh the advantages and disadvantages of the available options and make an informed decision.

I try not to rush when I'm negotiating a reduced fee with a new patient so I don't agree to something I might regret or resent in the future. At the beginning of each year, I estimate my required earnings for the following 12 months, and use these figures to calculate how much care I can reasonably provide at a reduced rate. After these slots are filled, I'll refer patients in need of subsidized treatment to other providers or to community clinics.

If the patient's financial situation changes, I'll renegotiate the fee at that time. Example 8.4 illustrates what I might do if I learn that a patient with a reduced fee could, in fact, pay full fee if she used financial assets reserved for "other expenses."

EXAMPLE 8.4

The therapist confronts a private practice patient receiving a reduced fee who has monetary resources that were kept secret

SALLIE: So, I just can't stand living in the dorm anymore. I think I might try to move into an apartment this summer. Maybe I'll live alone. I think the change would really decrease my stress level.

THERAPIST: When did you start to think about this?

SALLIE: Well, when I turned 21, I was able to access a trust fund from my grandparents for school and other stuff. I was thinking about it this week. I can actually afford to move out of student housing this year.

THERAPIST: What does the trust fund provide for you?

SALLIE: Well, it is for college expenses, and maybe a trip after graduation. I want to spend it carefully so maybe it can help me with a down payment on a house someday.

THERAPIST: Your financial situation has changed from when we originally set your reduced fee.

SALLIE: Not really. This money isn't supposed to be used for psychotherapy.

THERAPIST: When I agreed to the reduced fee, I indicated that we would renegotiate if your financial status improved. I'd like to raise the fee in accordance to our original discussion.

SALLIE: Well, my financial situation hasn't changed at all. Like I said, this money isn't for therapy but for living expenses.

THERAPIST: I understand that, but I also reserve my reduced fees for people who do not have adequate monetary resources. I am glad this money allows you some flexibility, but starting next month I will raise your fee to the rate of $100.00.

SALLIE: I don't know. That doesn't feel very fair to me, Dr. Bender.

THERAPIST: If I raised the fee to $100.00, how much of the money in the trust fund would you be using?

SALLIE: Not much, I guess. Just supplementing the $80.00 that I save each week to see you with $20.00 from the trust fund. But it just doesn't seem right.

THERAPIST: What if you were to spend the trust fund $20 on school expenses and pay the $20 for the therapy from other funds?

SALLIE: I never really thought of that and it would work, but I still think it feels really wrong.

THERAPIST: In what way?

SALLIE: I just worry what my parents would think about me using my trust fund for psychotherapy. Everyone—both sets of grandparents and my parents—saved years and years to give me this money.

THERAPIST: I can see that the trust fund carries a lot of feelings with it.

SALLIE: It really does. I feel so guilty about it.

THERAPIST: Guilty?

SALLIE: Well, my parents keep telling me how lucky I am to have a trust fund. It's supposed to help me pay for extra opportunities that they didn't have. I don't want to use it for therapy!

THERAPIST: How does your family view psychotherapy?

SALLIE: Even though I saw Dr. Anders in high school, they don't really understand what psychotherapy is. No one else has needed to see a shrink. And I've needed to talk to someone two times already and I'm only 21! Once should have been enough.

THERAPIST: I think this topic is worth talking about more. I will hold your fee at its lower rate this month, and we can discuss this in more depth. I will let you know about any potential fee decision at the end of this month before the next billing period begins.

SALLIE: Okay. But I feel really upset about this. Maybe I'll just need to stop therapy all together.

THERAPIST: I can see it bothers you very much. Why would you consider stopping altogether?

SALLIE: Well, like I said, if you increased my fee, I would have to use some of my trust fund money and I don't want to do that!

THERAPIST: To you, mixing the two—therapy and the trust fund—doesn't seem possible. Let's just try to understand this a little more together.

SALLIE: What's to understand? Like I told you, the trust fund was given to me under certain terms. It is supposed to be used for certain things, and therapy is not on the list!

THERAPIST: (*I notice a growing feeling of annoyance toward Sallie so I stay quiet, and only nod.*)

SALLIE: I don't know; this is just the way I feel.

THERAPIST: (*Regains composure.*) Is it a very strong feeling?

SALLIE: Yes, it is. So what are we going to do about it?

THERAPIST: For now, I think we should continue to talk about it.

In the next few sessions, Sallie continues to express her ambivalence about using her trust fund to subsidize her therapy. I wonder if I should keep her fee at the reduced rate, but I also know that I will feel very resentful treating Sallie at a reduced fee when she has the resources to pay my full fee. I consult with a trusted supervisor who wonders why my spouse, my child, and I should subsidize Sallie's therapy, and I decide to raise Sallie's fees during the next month of treatment. I tell Sallie about my decision two sessions prior to the one in which her fee will be raised.

Sallie starts the session by reviewing her week. Then, 10–15 minutes into the session, I interrupt.

THERAPIST: I want to hear more about your week, but I also wanted to let you know my decision about the fee today.

SALLIE: Oh, no. What did you decide to do?

THERAPIST: As I had mentioned earlier, this month will be at the previously decided lower fee. But, starting next month, I will be raising your fee to $100.00.

SALLIE: You are going to raise it? (*incredulous*)

THERAPIST: I am. Do you have strong feelings about this?

SALLIE: Umm . . . yes, I do!

THERAPIST: Can you tell me about them?

SALLIE: Well, I thought you understood. You must not understand me at all if you are going to raise my fee.

THERAPIST: I know there is a lot of emotion surrounding this issue. By raising your fee, which part don't I understand?

SALLIE: That my parents would be so upset if they knew about this, and my trust fund is an incredibly special gift. I can't use the money for something my parents wouldn't approve of!

THERAPIST: That doesn't feel like an option?

SALLIE: No! They'll think I'm so messed up that I need to spend this money on stupid therapy! (*Tears up and grabs a few tissues out of the box.*)

This illustrates how limit setting—holding to the frame—helps bring the underlying issues to the surface. Sallie may be more fearful of her parents' disapproving attitude than she is about the vague conditions of the trust fund.

THERAPIST: How will they feel you are messed up?

SALLIE: I'm incurable. I know they already think I'm nuts that I have to see a shrink to help me recover after a breakup with a boyfriend!

THERAPIST: Seeking help during a difficult time isn't seen as a strength?

SALLIE: No, it's not. And the fact that I tell you how I feel and you still increase my fee makes me really upset.

THERAPIST: Yes, I can see that the increase in fee is very upsetting to you.

SALLIE: So why did you have to do it?

THERAPIST: Because you are not as limited financially as I had previously believed.

SALLIE: Maybe I'll just stop therapy altogether.

THERAPIST: I would hope that wouldn't happen because of the fee increase, but it is always your choice. We have a lot to discuss about this loaded topic, and there is probably much to learn from it.

SALLIE: Yeah, but you aren't the one who is disappointing her parents.

THERAPIST: I'm beginning to understand how uncomfortable it would feel for you to disappoint your parents. Can you tell me more?

SALLIE: I think there was only one time that I spent money on something that they disapproved of. When I was in high school, I saved and saved my money for a really expensive CD Walkman. For whatever reason, they thought it was a stupid thing to buy. My mother said I was indulgent. She didn't understand why I wasn't happy with just a plain old radio or a tape player. But I love music and, for me, it was a great investment. Whenever I would get upset, I would listen on my headphones. I don't know. Sometimes my parents are strange about money.

THERAPIST: How do you feel now about your decision to get that CD player?

SALLIE: Umm, at the time I felt guilty, but now I feel that it was one of the best independent decisions that I have ever made.

THERAPIST: What allowed you to separate your own feelings from those of your parents?

SALLIE: I'm not sure. (*Pauses.*) I just knew I really needed it. It was a private safe place, sitting in my room senior year of high school and listening to my music. But I don't know if I feel as strongly about therapy.

THERAPIST: That's important to figure out. Perhaps it will help if you think about how life will be for you if you continued with psychotherapy and how it would be if you didn't.

SALLIE: I hadn't thought about it that way. I'm willing to give it some more thought, but are you still going to raise my fee?

THERAPIST: Yes, I am, for the reasons I explained, but I appreciate that you are really working hard here. By having these conversations, I think we will learn more about what money means to you and how your sense of your own worth is influenced by your parents.

For any fee change, it is useful to follow the steps demonstrated in Example 8.4: (1) The therapist lets the patient know she is considering raising the fee weeks ahead of time in order to get the patient's input. (2) The therapist reminds the patient of the fee increase before the next bill. (3) Even after the decision to increase the fee has been made, the therapist remains open to talking empathically, and not defensively, about the patient's monetary concerns.

BILLING

Unless a patient prefers to pay at each visit, I bill for my services at the end of each month, and expect payment within 30 days. A money exchange at every meeting can be distracting, so I only insist on session-to-session payment when a patient has repeatedly fallen behind on her account.

If I meet with a patient within the first week of a month, I'll hand the patient last month's bill at the beginning of our session. This direct interaction invites an immediate discussion of the bill if there are any problems or questions and clearly demonstrates that the billing process is an interaction between the patient and me. Some patients may experience the immediacy of this interaction as distracting and unempathic. If this is the case, I could encourage the patient to talk openly about her reaction. An in-depth discussion on this topic may ultimately lead to a greater understanding of other monetary issues in the patient's life.

Another option is to send the bill through the mail with the expectation that it will be paid within the month. This is Dr. Messner's preference. I also do this for patients I see infrequently, or for patients whose parents are paying for their treatment. With mailing, monetary issues do not interrupt the treatment unless payment isn't received.

I outline my billing method for a new patient during one of our first sessions. For most patients, a straightforward and clear discussion about monetary issues early in the treatment sets the stage for an unencumbered collection process. By explicitly outlining the method for money transfer, it is also easier to delve into any emotional reaction to the billing process.

Every now and then patients don't pay their bill, and the overdue balance becomes an issue within the psychotherapy. If Sallie did not pay her bill, and then took a break from therapy, I would send her duplicate bills over the next few months. Often, a second bill sent the month following the first one is all that is necessary to procure payment. If she still continues to have an outstanding balance, I would discuss the issue with her by phone, and would design a payment plan if she were struggling with limited financial resources. Until the balance is paid in full, I would continue to contact Sallie on a regular basis, either by phone or via a monthly statement noting the unpaid balance. As long as a patient works with me in good faith, I don't mind if the bill is paid off slowly. On the other hand, if the patient is unwilling to take any responsibility for her bill, I would eventually add this note to the bottom of one of her monthly statements: "If the payment in full is not received by MM/DD/YYYY, it will be referred for collection."

The situation becomes more complicated for the nonindigent patient who continues to come for appointments without paying her bill. The first time I was faced with a patient who didn't pay her bill, I didn't intiate any discussion about the unpaid balance and just hoped silently that the patient would eventually pay her outstanding balance. This strategy didn't work, and it even jeopardized the therapy as I became more and more resentful of the unpaid bill. In Example 8.5, Sallie has the financial resources to pay her bill, but her ambivalence about the therapeutic process impedes the payment process. The best approach combines business finesse with some psychotherapeutic principles.

EXAMPLE 8.5

Discussing payment with the patient who hasn't paid

It is December 29th, and Sallie has not paid for her November's sessions. The bill is due December 31.

THERAPIST: (*Interrupts flow of conversation about 15 minutes into the session.*) I definitely want to hear more about what has been going on, but we do need to take a few minutes to iron out a few administrative details.

SALLIE: Oh, like what?

THERAPIST: I wondered, how is it going with the bill?

SALLIE: Oops. I guess it's due really soon, huh? I don't think I'll be able to get you the check by the end of the month, but I'll definitely pay you next week. I just forgot. Thanks for reminding me.

By the next session, the bill is overdue. I interrupt Sallie at approximately the 15-minute mark.

THERAPIST: I wanted to make sure to ask you about the bill this session because it is overdue.

SALLIE: Oh no! Did I forget again? I don't know what is wrong with me! I'm so sorry, Dr. Bender.

THERAPIST: Maybe this is something we should be curious about. What do you think is making it hard to remember this?

SALLIE: Oh, I don't know. I feel so guilty that you have to keep reminding me, but then I keep forgetting to write the check before I leave home. I am really sorry.

THERAPIST: Let's talk about it a bit. How does it feel to be paying a therapist in the first place?

SALLIE: Fine. I want to pay you. I'm just disorganized; I'll make sure to bring the check next time.

Next Session

I bring up subject of money at the beginning of the session as the treatment is in jeopardy if the bill is not paid very soon.

THERAPIST: Let's start the session by touching base about the bill.

SALLIE: Umm, oh my goodness, I forgot my checkbook again. I don't know what is wrong with me. I am so embarassed.

THERAPIST: Let's also take some time to try to understand why the bill has been so difficult to pay. Are you in any financial trouble?

SALLIE: Well, things aren't great, but they aren't incredibly tight either. I just need to review my expenses to make sure I can pay you. I think I should be able to do it.

THERAPIST: How do you feel about continuing to forget to write me a check?

SALLIE: I don't know. I always try to remember after I leave here and then I forget.

THERAPIST: When you think about payment and money in therapy, what feelings come up?

SALLIE: I don't know. Money is hard for me.

THERAPIST: Hard for you in what way?

SALLIE: It just feels weird paying you to talk to me.

THERAPIST: I'm glad you could share this with me. Could you tell me any more about this weird feeling?

SALLIE: I'm not sure what it is exactly. It feels uncomfortable to pay you to listen to me.

THERAPIST: Can you tell me more about how it is uncomfortable?

SALLIE: I just feel that therapy is such a strange concept. We sit here and talk about all these very private things and then I get a bill weeks later. Why can't I make friends that would listen to me for free? Why am I so screwed up that I need to do this?

THERAPIST: Does part of you wish that I would be your friend rather than your psychotherapist?

SALLIE: Sort of . . .

THERAPIST: (Nods encouragingly.)

SALLIE: I just wonder how you view this whole thing.

THERAPIST: For the sake of the therapy, can you tell me what you imagine?

SALLIE: I don't know. I just sometimes wonder if you only care about the money. Therapy is pretty expensive. Maybe that is the only reason you do this.

THERAPIST: Can you tell me more?

SALLIE: I just worry that all your concern is fake. Maybe it is so hard for me to pay because that makes it crystal clear that that you are not a friend. And you are the nicest person I know at college right now. It feels so weird. Maybe if I don't pay you, I can sort of pretend that we have a connection that is more real.

THERAPIST: It doesn't feel real because it is a therapeutic relationship?

SALLIE: Yes, the money clouds it all.

THERAPIST: I can understand that this feeling might make it more difficult to pay. I hope we can understand it more together so the whole process will feel a bit easier for you. However, in order to continue working together, I will need to get payment for the sessions.

The Bill Payment Is 1 Month Late

SALLIE: Dr. Bender, I have your check! I am sorry it was so late. I'll pay for this session now too. It feels so good to be caught up.

THERAPIST: Considering the difficulties you had before, what enabled you to bring this check now?

SALLIE: I'm not sure really. I got a little worried that you might stop seeing me if I didn't manage to pay up soon.

Five Weeks Later, the Bill is 1 Week Late

THERAPIST: (*Brings up topic midsession.*): Let's take a few minutes to review the money situation. Twice now, your bill has been late, and to avoid a similar situation in the future, I think it would be reasonable for you to pay for each session at the time of the meeting—starting next week. What would be better for you—to pay at the beginning or at the end of each session? [*I provide two choices that are acceptable to me.*]

SALLIE: Oh, the end, I think. It might be hard to get started if I'm sitting here writing a check before the session starts.

THERAPIST: How do you feel about this arrangement?

SALLIE: I guess it's fine, but I can't start today. I'll pay for two sessions and last month's bill next week. Is that okay?

THERAPIST: That would be fine. I think it will be useful for us to have a regular payment schedule to follow.

SALLIE: You're probably right. I'll see you next week.

At the End of the Next Session

THERAPIST: We'll need to stop a couple of minutes early so I can give you the bill for this session.

SALLIE: Oh, yes. I am supposed to pay up today. I don't know how to say this, but I don't have my checkbook again. Now what should we do? I'm really sorry.

THERAPIST: I think we need to find a way for billing to work within the therapy, and then at some point, we will have the opportunity to try to understand more about what this means.

SALLIE: Dr. Bender, you know that I intend to pay the bill. I'm not trying to cheat you. I'll pay you next week.

THERAPIST: I'm glad that you plan to pay me next time, but, as I had mentioned before, I would like for us to have a dependable payment plan so you don't end up having a large outstanding bill like before. In the future, I hope we can talk more about some of the obstacles that are making it difficult for you to pay on a regular basis. Meanwhile I think that it is time for you pay me before each session. If you don't have your payment at the beginning of our next session, we'll reschedule the appointment. Does that sound reasonable to you?

SALLIE: No, I don't think that's fair.

THERAPIST: Considering what's been going on, what do you think is fair?

SALLIE: In another month, my finances will be in great shape, and it will be no problem to pay my balance, but right now I'm pinching pennies.

THERAPIST: I'm not willing to wait a month, but I am willing to extend your credit 1 week more. [*In other circumstances, I might be more willing to set up a payment plan when I hear a patient is struggling with her finances. In Sallie's case, she has not been responsible about her outstanding balance, so I only offer limited flexibility.*]

At the Beginning of the Next Session

THERAPIST: Before we begin, here is the bill for the last two sessions and today's meeting.

SALLIE: (*Searching anxiously through her backpack*) Oh no, oh, please don't be mad at me. Dr. Bender, I messed up again. I didn't bring my checkbook. What happens now? (*Begins to tear up.*)

THERAPIST: I am sorry, but, as I told you, I am not willing to work with you this hour with the outstanding bill. We can reschedule for another session, but in order to have that session, it will be necessary for you to pay your balance.

SALLIE: But Dr. Bender, what happens if there is an emergency and I need to talk to you?

THERAPIST: I hope that we can continue to work together after the bill is paid. Until then, in case of any type of emotional crisis, I recommend that you go to your local emergency room.

Sallie Gane is not allowed to continue the session, and I charge her for the adjourned session. She sends me a check in the mail to cover her balance. If she starts to forget her checkbook at future scheduled sessions, I would follow the same protocol that has been outlined here.

When Sallie repeatedly forgets her checkbook, we can assume that the action is multidetermined and emotionally meaningful. She is acting in a passive–aggressive manner when she repeatedly denies me payment but does not acknowledge the hostility driving this behavior. As the therapy deepens, Sallie and I may learn more about her use of delay and withholding in multiple personal relationships. As relationships rarely flourish in such an environment, Sallie's interactions with others might improve substantially when she is ready to learn about this part of herself.

When I have to withhold Sallie's treatment because of an unpaid bill, I make sure to inform her of the services available at her local emergency facilities in case of an emotional crisis. Any other approach provides therapy for free, and supports Sallie's wish that I treat her as a friend and without charge.

Nowadays, rather than watch the bill increase in parallel with my own internal resentment, I try to talk about unpaid balances early and often. I am more empathic at exploring the patient's feelings about monetary issues when only 1 month of treatment is overdue. Sometimes, the discussion is all that is needed to resolve the billing crisis so treatment can continue unhindered.

When all else fails for a patient with adequate financial resources who avoids paying her bill, it is time to consult a collection agency. Your supervisors will be able to recommmend a reputable business, and most medical, psychological, or other professional associations can also provide a list of ethical and decent collection agencies.

In some instances, a patient doesn't pay her bill because of financial difficulties. My response to the patient's needs will depend upon my financial limitations. I could help facilitate further treatment by reducing the patient's fee temporarily if I am able. I could also treat the patient on credit, or refer her to a subsidized clinic for continued treatment after working out a payment plan for her outstanding bill.

Now and then, a patient's parents refuse to pay the bill in a timely manner, after they have promised to subsidize the treatment. Example 8.6 illustrates some tactics I use when faced with this predicament.

EXAMPLE 8.6

How to react when a patient's relative refuses to subsidize the therapy as previously promised

In early December, I mail Sallie a bill for her November sessions. I know she will be forwarding it to her parents. The bill is still unpaid in early January.

Midsession, January 2nd

THERAPIST: I wanted to mention to you that I haven't received payment for the last bill that I sent to you. Are there any problems with the payment that you know about?

SALLIE: Umm, I'm really sorry I haven't paid it yet. I mailed it to my parents and they haven't mailed me back the payment yet.

THERAPIST: Any ideas why they haven't mailed you the payment yet?

SALLIE: I don't know really. I sometimes wonder what they think about the fact that I am in therapy again.

THERAPIST: What have you wondered about?

SALLIE: Oh, when they learned I was back in treatment, they made a couple stupid wisecracks about it. They couldn't understand why I needed a therapist to talk about a boy. According to my mom, I might as well call "rent-a-friend." But, after all the jokes, they did say that they would pay for the sessions.

THERAPIST: How did you feel when they referred to me as your "rent-a-friend?"

SALLIE: Horrible. Wouldn't you?

THERAPIST: Why would they hurt you like that?

SALLIE: I don't know. I'm probably being oversensitive.

THERAPIST: Have you discussed this bill with them?

SALLIE: Not really. I let them know it was in the mail, and I expected they would mail me back a check pretty quickly so I could pay you on time. I don't know what's wrong.

THERAPIST: Could I have your permission to call them about the bill?

SALLIE: Oh, I don't know. They'll pry for details about my life.

THERAPIST: I can understand your concern. How should we approach this so both the therapy and your privacy can be protected?

SALLIE: Let me talk to my parents one more time. I should have the check by next week.

THERAPIST: Okay, that should be fine.

Sallie comes to the next meeting in tears.

THERAPIST: (*Waits for Sallie to start talking.*)

SALLIE: My parents are acting so weird. They have all these excuses why they can't give me the check this week. I don't get it. They promised to support the therapy, and I know money isn't the issue. I don't know what to do.

THERAPIST: What was the conversation like?

SALLIE: When I asked about the check, they were very vague. I don't know if they plan to mail it anytime soon.

THERAPIST: Have they ever done something like this before?

SALLIE: Once when I asked them for some money to fund a school retreat to Vermont for the weekend, they said yes at first, but never came through with the money.

THERAPIST: Then what happened?

SALLIE: Well, eventually, they paid, but only after I talked to them about the project in more detail.

THERAPIST: Could that be what they are looking for here? Maybe if they feel more included in your treatment they would be more willing to pay. How would it feel to you if I gave them a call to try to clear things up?

SALLIE: (*sniffling*) Okay, but what are you going to tell them?

THERAPIST: That is an important question. Do you feel comfortable with me describing any piece of what we have been talking about?

SALLIE: You can tell them that I sometimes feel depressed.

THERAPIST: And may I fill them in on some of the symptoms of depression that you have experienced, like loss of sleep and appetite?

SALLIE: Yeah, that would be okay I guess.

THERAPIST: Anything that you would like me to avoid mentioning?

SALLIE: Don't tell them any details about Charlie and the whole problem with him. Are you going to tell them a lot about me?

THERAPIST: No, but I do think a bare-bones outline of what we are doing may help them understand the therapy a little better. Would you be willing to sign a form authorizing me to talk to them?

SALLIE: Okay.

THERAPIST: I will also fill you in on our conversation at our next meeting.

SALLIE: That sounds good.

Phone Call to Mr. and Mrs. Gane

THERAPIST: May I talk to Mr. or Mrs. Gane please?

MRS. GANE: This is Mrs. Gane.

THERAPIST: Hello, this is Dr. Bender, I am the psychiatrist treating your daughter, Sallie.

MRS. GANE: Oh, yes. Is Sallie okay?

THERAPIST: She has some difficulties, but I think treatment will help her feel better. I am calling to clarify whether you are willing to finance her therapy. Her current bill is overdue.

MRS. GANE: Of course we will provide whatever Sallie needs, but do you think she really needs therapy? Breakups are a normal part of growing up.

THERAPIST: I think therapy could be very helpful, as your daughter is suffering from symptoms of depression at this point.

MRS. GANE: Oh, I don't know. Sallie was already in therapy once during high school. I don't think she really needs any more.

She was doing just fine before the breakup with Charlie. She'll survive. I'm sure she'll be fine in a couple of months.

THERAPIST: There may be a misunderstanding. Your daughter has been struggling with some symptoms of depression, which is different from just having an unhappy mood. If it isn't treated, it can lead to other problems, some of them serious.

MRS. GANE: What kind of serious problems?

THERAPIST: When symptoms of a depression are untreated, a person can lose sleep and appetite, eventually become profoundly hopeless and, in about 15% of cases, become suicidal. If depression is treated, these problems are usually avoided.

MRS. GANE: Oh no! Is Sallie suicidal? Is that why you are calling?

THERAPIST: While I don't want to reveal the details of the therapy with Sallie, I can promise you that if I thought her condition was an emergency and she was at high risk for hurting herself, I would let you know.

MRS. GANE: Oh, that's a relief. Are there any less expensive clinics that could treat Sallie?

THERAPIST: There are some low-fee clinics in my area, but they often have waiting lists. Also, it can be difficult to start therapy with someone new if you had already started working closely with someone.

MRS. GANE: Dr. Bender, my son has some medical problems, and we seek second opinions all the time. It has never been an issue. He's been fine with switching doctors or seeing new people. Sallie might be upset at first, but I'm sure she would adjust to seeing someone at the school clinic. At least she could just meet a second therapist and see how it feels to talk to someone else.

THERAPIST: I would be glad to cooperate if she wishes to obtain a second opinion, but it is more complicated with psychotherapy than with other health professionals. It takes time to build trust to talk about emotionally intense issues. To start over can be very tough.

MRS. GANE: I am sorry, Dr. Bender, you do sound very concerned about my daughter, but I need to talk to my husband before I commit to paying for Sallie's treatment with you.

THERAPIST: Could you call me back by 5:00 P.M. tomorrow so I could also start talking about this dilemma with Sallie?

MRS. GANE: Sure, that shouldn't be a problem. I'll leave you a message.

THERAPIST: Okay, that would be very helpful.

Sallie's treatment is turning into a monetary morass. It isn't easy to figure out how to proceed. It would be difficult for her to switch providers at this point. For simplicity's sake, we'll say that her parents decide to support her treatment with me. In real life, it is equally possible that they might insist that she transfer her care to a clinic.

I would have several options if the Ganes refused to pay for Sallie's treatment because of financial constraints. As I review my personal financial situation, I can determine whether I can afford to accept a reduced fee or partially deferred fee from Sallie. If neither possibility is financially feasible, I could refer Sallie to a low-fee clinic for followup.

With a few preventive measures at the beginning of treatment, I might be able to avoid a situation like the one outlined in Example 8.6. Some therapists provide a patient with a form outlining payment procedures for the parents as soon as it is clear that the family will be responsible for the bill. The therapist's expectations are clear, and the parents are involved early, without disclosing personal information about the patient. A model form is provided at the end of this chapter. A similar form can be prepared for patients whose fees are deferred and who agree to pay at a future time. We have also provided an example of a bill for professional services.

Money is a complicated topic. At first, setting the fee, giving the bill, and then collecting payment may seem graceless and embarrassing to the beginning therapist. With experience, talking openly about monetary issues might be enlightening to the therapist and to the patient. Both individuals will benefit as they learn to grapple with these issues and their underpinnings in everyday life.

Key words: billing, collections, fee setting, free care, health insurance, managed care, negotiation, payment agreement, third-party payers

Payment Agreement for Treatment of a Relative or Acquaintance

I, _____, agree to pay Dr. _____

for professional services provided by him/her to _____,

my _____ (relationship), based on the following fee

schedule: _____.

Signed: _____

Date: _____

Witness: _____

Sample Bill for Services

Suzanne Bender, MD   Psychiatrist

258 Avenue of the Americas   [voice mail number]
Brookline, MA 02146   [pager number]

Sallie Gane

[address]

For Professional Services:

Diagnosis: Adjustment Disorder with Depressed Mood (309.0)

Date	Description	CPT Code	Charges
9/5/01	50-minute psychotherapy	90807	100.00
9/12/01	50-minute psychotherapy	90807	100.00
9/17/01	50 minute psychotherapy	90807	100.00

Previous balance:

Received:

Total charges:

Amount due: $300.00

State License Number: _____

9

Telephone Calls

From Dependencies to Emergencies

Phone calls during the course of a psychotherapy can range from ordinary scheduling communications, to emergencies that require a rapid assessment and definitive response, to repeated unnecessary contacts that may herald a regressive dependency. The therapist's responsibility is to discern the nature of the call and to respond appropriately. When responding to a phone call from a patient in crisis, the therapist needs to keep cool under pressure and to listen with empathy and respect. The goal is to help the patient access her most effective coping skills.

Every time I examined a patient in medical school, my work was checked and double-checked by physicians with more experience. I had a little more autonomy as a medical intern the year after graduation, but not much. As the physician on the inpatient team with the least amount of experience, I was responsible for the patient-care tasks that required the most time and the least skill. My beeper was my constantly intruding nemesis. Every time I received a new page, I knew that my job list for the day had just lengthened.

Internship does have some hidden perks that I didn't appreciate at the time. Because I didn't have primary responsibility for the patients on the ward, I was allowed to sign out all of my outstanding tasks after my call-shift was completed. Most of the time I was at everyone's beck and call, but when I was off, I was unreachable and free.

After internship, I began 3 years of residency training in adult psychiatry at Massachusetts General Hospital (MGH). I was ready to discard my role as the medical team's peon and to assume my new identity

134

as a novice psychiatrist, but I expected to be coddled as the ignorant newcomer.

I wasn't.

Instead, my training program highly valued early independence. While the entire staff, from the chief of psychiatry down, was always available for questions and for teaching, I was expected to grow out of my underling's mentality and to assume primary responsibility for my outpatients.

Within the first weeks of my residency, I became the designated psychiatrist for a small group of outpatients from the psychotherapy and psychopharmacology clinic. In case of an emergency, these patients (MY patients!) could page me through the hospital operator at any time. Except for vacations, for which I would organize coverage, I was expected to keep my beeper on from the moment I signed my employment papers until the day I graduated.

At first, I hated this arrangement. To be honest, I spent my first week at MGH trying to drum up support for an alternate emergency coverage system. At neighboring psychiatric programs, the residents signed their beepers out to the psychiatrist-on-call after 6:00 P.M. I expected that my colleagues would also want to adopt a less demanding coverage approach, but I was outvoted.

As I slowly adapted to the idea that my beeper was a new constant in my life, my next response, and my next mistake, was to romanticize my new appendage. Early on, I had only a few patients, so I didn't expect that I would be called frequently after-hours. I made sure the beeper was at my bedstand every night so I could respond immediately if it sounded its alarm. The arrangement became problematic as I began to view my beeper as a type of baby monitor. I was poised for the first "cry," ready to comfort and to help if my patient needed me.

While my attitude was steeped in empathic good intentions, it wasn't therapeutic. Patients aren't babies, and thinking and treating them as such is infantilizing.

It's a delicate issue. My patients should be able to reach me in a timely manner for questions and concerns. On the other hand, if I respond immediately and eagerly to nonemergency pages after-hours, I might encourage these types of interactions and even promote a patient's regression.

Patients first learn about a therapist's emergency availability at the beginning of a treatment. The verbal and nonverbal cues during this discussion can set the tone for the entire therapy. Early on, I unwittingly encouraged increased dependency by presenting the beeper (or the message center) as a conduit for unlimited after-hour contact.

EXAMPLE 9.1

The therapist sets herself up for abuse of her pager and of her emergency services.

End of First Consultation Session

THERAPIST: Let me tell you how to reach me in case you need to reschedule or in case of an emergency.

SALLIE: Okay.

THERAPIST: (*somewhat proudly*) I have my voice mail number listed on the card if you want to leave me a message. I also have my beeper on 24 hours a day in case of emergencies.

SALLIE: (*Nods.*)

THERAPIST: If you have an emergency, please page me immediately, and I will get back to you right away.

Without some clear limits, my statement "If you have an emergency, please page me immediately and I will get back to you right away" offers my pager as a patient's life line. Putting aside the fact that this statement may detrimentally affect my private life, acting as a personal 911 service can lead to disastrous consequences if modern technology fails, and a page transmission or reception is impaired. It would be tragic to miss the emergency page from a suicidal patient who is poised to act.

In Example 3.5, we reviewed how to talk to a new patient about the appropriate use of an emergency contact system. Whether I use a beeper, an answering service, or a voice mail system for emergency coverage, the basic rules are the same. I don't promise that I will be able to answer a message immediately, but I will return the call as soon as I can. A patient needs to know that it is her responsibility to go the nearest emergency room for acute intervention if she can't wait for my reply. From the get-go, the patient and I share the responsibility of reacting to a crisis.

Some therapists work in group practices or community clinics in which a designated person or a designated emergency facility takes calls after hours. For these patients, emergency care is provided by the clinician on call, who may or may not be the patient's primary provider. If a patient expresses disappointment that you, her personal therapist, won't be available after hours, her feelings should be thoroughly discussed within the treatment. But, usually the coverage system should not—and often cannot—be altered. To provide the most seamless coverage, each therapist in the group practice may want to inform her colleagues about her more fragile patients.

Surprisingly, although I graduated from my residency a few years ago, I've decided to stick with the beeper coverage system that I used in training. In retrospect, I appreciate that my training program didn't let me off the hook after hours. I've learned how to respond effectively to emergency pages and to set limits when a patient pages me excessively and inappropriately. There are advantages to this system that I hadn't recognized when it was first introduced to me. My pager is only available to my patients, and I am best prepared to answer their questions and to respond to their concerns because I know them so well. Since I am familiar with the personality style of each patient I treat, I am less likely to over- or to underreact to an emergency call.

My skill emerged slowly with experience. The following examples document some of the clinical scenarios that helped me learn to set limits with the patients in my practice.

DEPENDENCY PHONE CALLS

Early on, it was easy to let a phone call develop into an unscheduled therapy minisession.

EXAMPLE 9.2

The therapist allows and then encourages extended phone calls outside the session

On Wednesday, Sallie Gane cancelled an appointment for the first time on the morning of the appointment. She said she had "the flu" and was unable to come to our session.

On Saturday evening at the local movie theater with my husband, my beeper goes off. The beeper reads, "Sallie—" and is followed by her home phone number. She has never paged me before so I feel worried, leave the film, and head to a private area to call her back on my cell phone.

THERAPIST: May I talk to Sallie Gane please?

SALLIE: It's me. (*Sniffles.*) Dr. Bender, I just feel horrible, so I called you.

THERAPIST: What's wrong?

SALLIE: Well, remember I told you that one of the ways I have coped with the breakup with Charlie is to talk to my friend Gwen? Well, I just got in a terrible fight with her, and she is one of my only friends here at school. We were arguing about what to do tonight, and then, in the middle of the discussion, she got up and walked right out of my apartment. She even slammed the door. I don't know what to do. I'm sure she hates me now.

THERAPIST: How are you feeling?

SALLIE: I just feel overwhelmed. I didn't know what to do so I called you.

THERAPIST: Could you tell me what happened?

SALLIE: Well, it started over breakfast yesterday. (*Starts describing the details of the fight.*)

Sallie and I talk for 30 minutes. I miss the end of the movie. She receives a free psychotherapy minisession.

SALLIE: Oh, Dr. Bender, I feel so much better. I really appreciate that you called me back. You are the best doctor I have ever had!

THERAPIST: I'm glad I could help. Feel free to call me back if I can be of further help. [*I feel proud and accomplished that Sallie's crisis has passed due to my therapeutic intervention.*]

As an insecure novice practitioner, flush with the power of being a therapist rather than a medical intern, I believed that Example 9.2 modeled the ultimate empathic response. Sallie had felt abandoned and bereft, and I was available, approachable, and comforting. But Sallie's call was not truly an emergency clinical situation. She called for comfort, and I sacrificed a substantial amount of free time to take care of her. The question is whether this type of behavior should be encouraged.

There are many hazards to providing extensive psychotherapeutic discussions outside the scheduled session. If Sallie realizes that she can obtain an unscheduled evening minisession after an emotionally difficult day, this sort of phone call may be just the first in an upcoming series. Weekend or evening calls, especially after a missed weekly appointment, may become more frequent. Sallie might even try to substitute telephone calls for regular office visits. Complex payment problems might arise. If I'm really unlucky, the behavior might be contagious, with the patient's relatives or friends starting to call me to partake of my cost-free and—for them—"risk-free" therapy.

I might also become resentful of Sallie if she phones frequently. Without noticing, I might emotionally withdraw from her during our normally scheduled time, and the therapy itself might suffer. (Such a withdrawal would be an example of a countertransference enactment.)

Finally, by missing a significant amount of my planned evening entertainment in order to untangle Sallie's tiff with Gwen, I may convey the subtle message that I don't believe Sallie can cope with her troubles independently. If Sallie is treated as though she is incapable of handling basic crises without intervention, she might learn to fulfill these expectations. (This would be an example of intersubjectivity.)

However, we are not advocating a harsh response to a patient's page. Example 9.3 outlines how a therapist can be available while simultaneously setting limits and not encouraging evening/weekend comfort calls.

EXAMPLE 9.3

Assessment of a situation after a page followed by a quick but empathic crisis intervention

Same scene: Sallie pages me Saturday night while I am at the movies after she missed her appointment the Wednesday prior because of "the flu."

THERAPIST: May I talk to Sallie Gane please?

SALLIE: Well, remember. . . . [*See Example 9.2 for details of Sallie's fight with Gwen.*] What am I going to do?

THERAPIST: (*Assessing whether the situation is an emergency.*) How are you doing?

SALLIE: I feel so upset. I didn't know what to do, so I called you.

THERAPIST: It sounds like it was a difficult situation.

SALLIE: Yes, I can't believe it. She never walked out on me before. What if our friendship is totally over and done with?

THERAPIST: Have you ever gotten into these types of fights with Gwen before?

SALLIE: Yeah, we do tend to disagree. But this fight felt much more intense.

THERAPIST: I don't know a lot about your friendship with Gwen, but it does sound very troubling. We'll be able to discuss this situation with the time it deserves at our next session. Could you write down everything that happened so we can discuss it together on Wednesday?

SALLIE: Okay, but right now, I feel so overwhelmed.

THERAPIST: (*Continues calm, but firm tone.*) I think your first goal at this time is to take good care of yourself. At other times when you've been upset, what has been most soothing?

SALLIE: I don't know. Sometimes I feel a little better if I just veg out and watch TV. I guess sometimes I also write in my journal.

THERAPIST: Sounds good.

SALLIE: Well, my weekend has gotten off to a fabulous start (*sarcastically*), but I should be okay. Can you give me any advice about Gwen?

THERAPIST: I don't think there is an easy answer, but together on Wednesday we'll try to make some sense of what happened. (*with a tone of voice that I am starting to end the conversation*)

SALLIE: Thank you for calling. I'm sorry I bothered you.

THERAPIST: It sounds like a distressing situation, but I look forward to talking to you more about it on Wednesday. If you'd like, you can also share with me what you write in your journal.

SALLIE: Okay.

THERAPIST: See you Wednesday.

SALLIE: Bye, I'll see you on Wednesday.

As a page from Sallie is an unusual occurrence, I assess whether her call is a true emergency at the beginning of our conversation. If I were the least bit unsure of the severity of Sallie's crisis, or if I didn't know Sallie well, I would screen for suicidality during this phone call, even if it felt overprotective. Since I know Sallie fairly well at this point in the treatment, I know that her risk of self-harm after a fight with a friend is very low. She has no history of self-mutilatory behavior, severe substance abuse, or suicidal gestures. Since Sallie is not in imminent danger, I limit our conversation to a brief empathic crisis intervention.

At the beginning of the phone call, I make a conscious effort to validate Sallie's feelings. Then, as it would be impossible to review the fight in adequate detail over the phone without supporting the Saturday night paging behavior and ruining my weekend movie night, I postpone a more detailed discussion until our upcoming session. The comment "We'll be able to discuss this situation with the time it deserves at our next session" establishes the limits of the phone call while simultaneously acknowledging Sallie's concerns.

During our conversation, I avoid asking Sallie for any emotional associations to the upsetting episode. Instead I help her identify adaptive strategies that may enable her to feel a little better and enhance her independence. I don't take on the role as the primary comforting person in her life, and I avoid any invitation to call me later if she continues to feel upset.

By returning Sallie's page, reminding her of our upcoming session, and then encouraging recall of other ways she can comfort herself, Sallie's isolation is diminished; a malignant regression is not encouraged; and my private time is protected—all in a 5–10 minute phone call. In our subsequent session, I'll ask Sallie how she experienced our phone conversation. A discussion of her reaction will help increase my understanding of her predicament and will reinforce the therapeutic alliance.

A small percentage of patients try to contact me frequently between sessions. With a persistent, intransigent caller, I end each phone session as quickly as courtesy will allow and then discuss the calls in careful exploratory detail with the patient during the next scheduled session. If the number of nonemergency phone calls at inopportune times continue, I might be at risk for unleashing my frustration on the patient after enduring numerous interruptions. Instead, I limit my availability for nonemergency phone calls using the empathic, firm, and effective approach illustrated in Example 9.4.

EXAMPLE 9.4

Setting limits empathically for outside phone contact between sessions

Sallie has called me five nights in a row to talk about her troubles with Gwen.

Twenty Minutes into the Session Following the Calls

SALLIE: And so I just don't know what to do with Gwen!

THERAPIST: I do think we need to continue trying to understand this friendship and what it means to you, but I think it's important to take a little time to talk about your calls to me this week.

SALLIE: Oh, you were really helpful. Thank you for being there for me. This has been such a tough week.

THERAPIST: I'm glad I was helpful, but the best way to cope with an ongoing problem that is difficult to deal with—like Gwen—is to have a number of strategies in place that can help you feel better. Let's think together of other ways you've been able to soothe yourself when you've been upset in the past.

SALLIE: Well, I don't know. What do you mean?

THERAPIST: Before we started working together, what would you do to help yourself feel better when you felt upset?

SALLIE: I don't know . . . sometimes I would watch TV.

THERAPIST: (*Nods.*) What else?

SALLIE: Well, sometimes I would call my mother. She tends to get impatient, but sometimes she listens when I'm upset, and then I feel better.

THERAPIST: What other activities help? Have you ever tried writing in a journal?

SALLIE: I used to do that, but I haven't written anything for a long time. Do you think that might help?

THERAPIST: Journals are often very useful for helping someone think about a personal problem and how to approach it. I think these three things—watching TV, calling your mother, and writing in a journal—could be a good preliminary list to comfort you during this tough time with Gwen. How does it feel to you?

SALLIE: I don't know. I guess I could do these things when I'm upset, but it really does help a lot to talk to you when I feel really overwhelmed.

THERAPIST: What is helpful about it?

SALLIE: Just touching base, I guess. Just hearing your voice helps.

THERAPIST: Can you tell me what is helpful about hearing my voice?

SALLIE: I just have been feeling so alone and upset this week. I just feel a bit better after we talk. Otherwise, I feel totally alone.

THERAPIST: It does sound like it has been an especially painful week. Other than paging me, what would be some other options that might be helpful?

SALLIE: I don't know. . . .

THERAPIST: I have some ideas. Let me know what you think. If it is hearing my voice that is helpful, you could leave a message on my voice mail when you are feeling lonely, and we can discuss the message at our next meeting.

SALLIE: Oh, I'd feel stupid doing that.

THERAPIST: How come?

SALLIE: Talking to a machine . . . I don't know. It might help, but it wouldn't make me feel that much better. I need to hear you talk back.

THERAPIST: Have you ever imagined what I might say at such a time? [*I'm trying to help Sallie conjure up an internal image of me for comfort between sessions so she won't need to call me after each disappointment. This is an example of evocative memory.*]

SALLIE: No.

THERAPIST: What if you try it now?

SALLIE: Huh? How?

THERAPIST: Do you remember how you felt before you called me last night?

SALLIE: No, this feels stupid. I just need some extra support right now. Talking to you helps with that, not just talking to your machine.

THERAPIST: I understand that the phone calls are helpful, but I'm not always available. With a whole group of comforting strategies, you're less likely to become dependent on talking to me to feel better.

SALLIE: (*Nods.*) I understand, I think. But if it helps me the most to talk to you, what is so bad about continuing our talks?

THERAPIST: I'm glad our talks are helpful, but the helpfulness doesn't last. If we can work together to help you find some coping strategies that will stay with you, your pain will decrease gradually. You'll also feel more confident in your ability to take care of yourself.

SALLIE: That makes sense, but I have so much to tell you. I sometimes forget to tell you everything during this meeting, so I call you to fill you in.

THERAPIST: I am interested in being filled-in, but therapy works best if we try to concentrate the work we do together during scheduled sesssions. Since this is a crisis-filled week, would it be useful to meet an extra time?

SALLIE: Maybe. . . .

THERAPIST: What would that be like for you?

SALLIE: I think it might help to talk about this some more. It feels like the one session a week is up before it has even started.

THERAPIST: Should we schedule an extra session this week?

SALLIE: I think it's a good idea. Let's do that.

THERAPIST: Let's also plan together how you can help yourself feel better if you have another difficult evening sometime this week.

SALLIE: Yeah. What should I do?

THERAPIST: What if you try writing down your thoughts, phoning your mother, watching TV, or calling my voice mail between the two sessions? If you are feeling that the situation is really an emergency and cannot wait, you can page me. If I don't answer right away and you feel you need to talk to someone immediately, it is important not to sit and wait but to go straight to the nearest emergency room.

SALLIE: I don't get it. I wouldn't feel comfortable going to an emergency room. Why would I go there?

THERAPIST: If for whatever reason you felt that you were in danger of hurting yourself in any way, that would be a reason to hightail it to the nearest ER. If you were in danger, I would want you to get immediate care in that instance and not just wait around for me to call you back. [*I reinforce the idea that my pager is really for emergencies only.*]

SALLIE: Oh, I have never felt that bad. I don't think you have to worry about that.

THERAPIST: I'm glad. But it is good to review together how to use the voice mail and beeper so we both know how to approach an emergency.

SALLIE: Okay. I'm sorry if I beeped you too much this week.

THERAPIST: I think it's useful that we talked about it. This new approach will actually serve you better than if we continued to talk every night. The two sessions will provide some increased support. With fewer phone calls, you'll also learn how to help yourself feel better when I'm not readily available.

SALLIE: It feels a little scary, but it makes sense.

If I set limits before I've become frustrated with a patient's repeated calls, I'm much more empathic and able to follow the calm, firm approach outlined here. By supporting Sallie's nonregressive coping mechanisms (methods of comforting herself that don't involve talking to me on the phone), I play to her emotional strengths. When Sallie expresses her need to talk to me more often, the extra session is a viable alternative that works within the limits of my schedule and the frame of her treatment.

As a trainee, one of my supervisors told me about a patient who would not respond to any clear restrictions, such as those outlined in Example 9.4. Despite frequent attempts at limit setting by all of his care providers, including his primary care doctor and various specialists, he paged them all frequently and at all hours whenever he became upset. To limit the patient's spiraling regression, his psychiatrist wrote a letter with the help and approval of the hospital's legal department. The letter was signed by all clinicians involved in the patient's care.

The letter outlined that the patient was not allowed to page any providers at any time if he wanted to continue to receive medical care at the hospital. Instead, frequent brief meetings with all of his clinicians were provided. All emergency care was referred to the hospital's emergency room. If the patient did page any of his clinicians, the practioners were legally obligated to respond, but then, as documented in the letter, they could refer him to another facility for further treatment.

The psychiatrist on this multidisciplinary team presented the letter to his patient. He stated that the medical team was concerned about the patient's continued welfare and had outlined what care they could and couldn't provide rather than just "refer" his care elsewhere, as had happened at numerous other hospitals. Since the therapist's resentment was held in check by the letter's protective limit setting, the document could be presented with consideration and concern, rather than with exasperation and desperation.

The psychiatrist was surprised by the patient's response. The patient viewed the letter as a caring gesture. It served as both a communication of treatment limits and a tangible memento of the hospital staff's interest in his condition. He carried it in his billfold for months. The serial pages ceased.

COPING MECHANISMS FOR THE THERAPIST: HOW TO DEAL WITH FRUSTRATION

As patients tested my limits, I needed to find ways to release my frustration without affecting the treatment detrimentally. As a medical student, I imagined that once I became a psychiatrist I would always feel calm and contained when working with patients. In reality, even after years of experience, I sometimes feel irritated when faced with emotionally difficult clinical situations. The trick is figuring out how to release my frustration in an effective way that still spares my patient.

My first stop is often with supervisors and colleagues. To stay in close touch with the psychotherapy community, I continue to pay for intermittent supervision and to attend a peer supervision group once a month. When grappling with complicated clinical scenarios, the mutual support makes all the difference.

I've also used directed fantasy to release frustration. This established technique works best if the fantasy is affect-laden, detailed, and intense. If I'm furious at a patient, an uncivilized fantasy may be a very effective way to manage my feelings. In my head, I can express my frustration freely. When the distinction between fantasy and action is clearly delineated, there is no harm in releasing anger in any imaginary scenario.

Such procedures are well documented in the cognitive-behavioral therapy literature.

Once I've expressed my anger in a forum apart from my patient, her treatment will be protected from intense unprocessed irritation. By releasing pent-up patient-evoked hostility, I also will be protecting my family, friends, and associates from emotional spillovers of work-related emotions.

A therapy may even benefit if the therapist is aware of an unsavory countertransference reaction toward a patient. If I'm aggravated by a patient, I'm probably not the first person to feel this way toward her, but I may be the first person able to talk to her about her actions in an empathic and curious manner. After privately pinpointing my patient's behaviors that are evoking my anger, I try to understand what benefit she might be deriving from these actions. Probably she wouldn't be acting in this manner unless it satisfied some type of internal—perhaps unconscious—need. Maybe over time the two of us will be able to understand the motivation fueling her behavior. That understanding might eventually enable the patient to improve her relationships with me and with others.

EMERGENCY PHONE CALLS

Fortunately, the true psychiatric emergency is a relatively rare event, but it does happen. About 30,000 completed suicides occur in the United States yearly. A phone conversation with an actively suicidal patient is an anxiety-provoking experience for even the most experienced clinicians.

EXAMPLE 9.5

Emergency evaluation by phone

I receive a page from Sallie Gane on Saturday evening at 7:00. Sallie has not paged me previously.

THERAPIST: May I talk with Sallie Gane please?

SALLIE: Dr. Bender, thanks for calling back. (*muffled, tearful voice*)

THERAPIST: You sound upset. Can you tell me what's happened?

SALLIE: I don't know. I can't really talk about it, but I just can't stand it anymore!

THERAPIST: What do you mean?

SALLIE: I'm not sure, but I thought I would call you before I did something stupid.

THERAPIST: I am glad you called me. What were you thinking of doing?

SALLIE: I don't know. I wish I could just go to sleep and escape.

THERAPIST: I'm concerned; you must be feeling pretty desperate. Have you made any plans to make this "escape"?

SALLIE: Well, I just went to the drugstore. . . .

THERAPIST: What did you get?

SALLIE: I bought a bunch of stuff. Umm . . . some pain relievers, some sleeping pills.

THERAPIST: Are you planning to take them?

SALLIE: Maybe. Everybody hates me—Charlie, Gwen. I thought this would just make me feel better, but I thought I would call you first.

THERAPIST: I am really glad that you did. Let's think together what we can do now to help you.

SALLIE: I just feel so horrible!

THERAPIST: What would be helpful to you?

SALLIE: I'm not sure. . . .

THERAPIST: How safe do you feel tonight?

SALLIE: Ummm, what do you mean?

THERAPIST: Well, for starters, are you in a familiar place? Are you at home?

SALLIE: Yes, I'm in my room.

THERAPIST: Is anyone there with you?

SALLIE: No. I'm here alone.

THERAPIST: I wonder if you will be okay at your apartment alone overnight, or if it would be better for you to be seen in an emergency room tonight if you are at risk of hurting yourself.

SALLIE: I'm not sure.

THERAPIST: If you are not sure, then I think we should be extra careful and have you come to an emergency room to be evaluated.

SALLIE: Oh, I don't know if I want to go in. It's so cold out tonight!

THERAPIST: Here are our options. We could set up a time for you to check in with me by phone tomorrow as well as a special meeting on Monday to talk together or you can go in tonight to see someone. I can call and let them know to expect you.

SALLIE: Then someone I've never talked to before would want to know what's bothering me?

THERAPIST: Yes, but he or she could call me as well to learn a little background.

SALLIE: I think I'd rather just see you on Monday.

THERAPIST: Do you think you will make it through the night without hurting yourself?

SALLIE: Yes, I guess so. . . .

THERAPIST: "I guess so" doesn't feel safe enough for me. If you are unsure, I think you need to be seen tonight.

SALLIE: Well, I still feel depressed, but it does help to know that I have an appointment with you on Monday.

THERAPIST: Where are the pills?

SALLIE: On my desk.

THERAPIST: What about flushing them down the toilet?

SALLIE: Are you serious?

THERAPIST: Very. If you aren't going to the ER, we need to make sure you are 100% safe tonight.

SALLIE: Okay, I'll do it.

THERAPIST: Why don't I stay on the phone while you do it right now?

SALLIE: Wow, you take this stuff so seriously!

THERAPIST: I really do.

SALLIE: Okay, hold on.

THERAPIST: Yes, of course. [*I can hear the toilet flushing in the background.*]

SALLIE: Dr. Bender?

THERAPIST: I'm here. Did you flush the pills?

SALLIE: Yes.

THERAPIST: All of them?

SALLIE: Yes.

THERAPIST: How are you feeling now?

SALLIE: Better since you called.

THERAPIST: But still pretty awful?

SALLIE: Yes.

THERAPIST: One other thing: Would you tell me your address?

SALLIE: Why do you want to know?

THERAPIST: I don't have your record with me. I want to know where you are just in case I would need to send help at some point.

SALLIE: Oh, Dr. Bender, what do you mean? You wouldn't send the police over or something, would you?

THERAPIST: At this point, I feel good about our plan to touch base tomorrow and then meet on Monday, but I think it is important that I have your address available in case things were to get worse.

SALLIE: Okay, I guess. I'm at 1111 Central Street in downtown Boston.

THERAPIST: How are you feeling as we continue to talk?

SALLIE: Still pretty upset.

THERAPIST: How are the thoughts of hurting yourself right now?

SALLIE: Well, they still cross my mind.

THERAPIST: Thoughts are troubling enough, but the real question is whether you have any intention of acting on them.

SALLIE: No, I really don't think so.

THERAPIST: What if the plan to hurt yourself returns in the middle of the night or tomorrow?

SALLIE: I don't know . . . I'll call you?

THERAPIST: Yes, page me or go straight to the emergency room.

SALLIE: Okay, thanks.

THERAPIST: You are very welcome. Now, would you page me as a check-in at 10:00 A.M. tomorrow and come to the office at 3:00 on Monday?

SALLIE: Let me check my book. . . . Yep, I can do both of those.

THERAPIST: Until our meeting, what will you do to comfort yourself?

SALLIE: I think I'll call this girl, Nancy, who I met in my journalism class and ask her if she could spend the day with me tomorrow. I'd feel better if I had some company.

THERAPIST: What if Nancy isn't available?

SALLIE: I guess I'll just go to the library then. There's a table where the economics students study together. Maybe I'll see someone I know from class there.

THERAPIST: I think that is a very good plan. What are your plans for tonight?

SALLIE: I'm pretty tired now. I think I'll just go to bed soon. I feel better than when I called you.

THERAPIST: I'm glad. I look forward to talking to you tomorrow at 10 A.M. and seeing you on Monday at 3:00 P.M. [*establishing a future*]

SALLIE: At your office?

THERAPIST: Yes. I'll be waiting for you.

SALLIE: Thank you. I'll be there. [*confirming a future, an essential feature in estimating safety*]

A suicidal crisis is a psychiatric emergency that must be evaluated thoroughly and immediately. In Example 9.5, I assess Sallie's suicidal risk by reviewing her suicidal ideation, intent, and plan. I devise my treatment strategy based on her current risk profile and her degree of cooperation.

Sallie has two risk factors for suicide: major depressive disorder and an interpersonal loss. In addition, it is particularly worrisome that she has a predefined plan and has taken some steps to enact it. It is reassuring that she called me before taking the pills, because this shows some forethought, restraint, and a wish for help. During the phone evaluation, she is engageable, honest, and cooperative, so I feel comfortable postponing the face-to-face assessment until Monday.

In an emergency clinical situation, I don't limit my phone availability. Instead, I invite Sallie to contact me during the night or the following day if her suicidality increases. While our planned phone check-in will provide some extra support on Sunday morning, I still try to encourage emotional growth rather than regression by helping Sallie think of activities that would comfort her during the rest of the weekend. I try to discern how much she is willing and able to accomplish for the sake of her own safety.

If I had any reason to believe Sallie was lying to me and had already taken the pills, or if Sallie had refused to go the emergency room for further evaluation but had also been unable to contract for safety convincingly, I would be forced to call her local police department to escort her to the nearest emergency room against her will. With the possibility of overdose or other self-harm, I could also arrange to send an ambulance. If I didn't have her address or if she refused to give it to me, the police could access her address from her telephone number. Sending Sallie to an emergency room against her will would probably cause at least a temporary rift in our therapeutic alliance, but that would be preferable to the dangers of postponing urgent treatment.

Some patients are at higher risk for self-harm than others. Men in the United States are at higher risk than women for completed suicides, although women may attempt suicide more frequently. (The reverse is true in China and in some other countries.) Patients with a chronic medical illness such as AIDS, substance abuse, major depression, severe panic disorder, borderline personality disorder, impulsiveness, and history of violence, trauma, or psychosis are all at higher risk for completed suicide. Life stressors, including advanced age (especially older men), adolescence, divorce, bereavement, or loss of employment, are also associated with suicide attempts. A review of a patient's risk factors helps guide my assessment, but ultimately I evaluate each patient's specific situation apart from statistical risk factors.

Very early in my psychiatric training, only 3 months after my internship, one of my former patients from the adult psychiatric inpatient unit overdosed and died 8 weeks after discharge. During her 12-week hospitalization, the patient had been treated with electroconvulsive therapy (ECT) for a malignant psychotic depression. At the time of discharge, she had been hopeful and future-oriented, although still vulnerable due to the severity of her disease. She had close followup scheduled with her caring and competent outpatient provider. The attending psychiatrist on the inpatient unit and I tried to piece together what had happened. We were shocked and so sad. She was only 32.

Even though I wasn't this patient's primary psychiatrist, I still felt completely overwhelmed and guilt-ridden when I heard the news. During our first year of psychiatric training, Dr. Messner had mentioned that at least one member of my class might have a patient successfully commit suicide in the next 12 months. I had been sure that I would be spared, and I was wrong.

For months after this young woman's suicide, I obsessed about my suicidality assessments whenever a patient mentioned any thoughts of self-harm. During an evaluation, I would repeatedly ask a patient about her suicidal thoughts, intent, and plan. I began to worry that my evaluations were too lengthy or too anxiety-driven and consulted with Dr. Messner. I remember exactly what he said, even though the conversation occurred over 7 years ago. "Take as much time as you need, Suzanne," he said. "Review your suicidality assessment as many times as you'd like in order to feel comfortable with your treatment decision." This is the wisdom I would like to impart to you. If you are unsure about the patient's safety, keep talking to him or her in detail until you feel confident about his or her safety or the need to hospitalize. There is no need to rush these types of evaluations. Take your time to feel comfortable with your decision. The patient's survival may be at stake.

Over time (and after making many of the mistakes outlined in this chapter), I've learned how to provide intersession and emergency care effectively. Because I have followed the strategies we have provided in this chapter, my patients now rarely page me after 6:00 P.M., and I am awakened at night by a page only a few times a year. This isn't because I have the most stable office practice in Boston, but because I have learned slowly how to help my patients maximize their coping skills and take advantage of our time together in the office, rather than to depend on evening or weekend phone or beeper contact for support. All these strategies are designed to prevent self-injurious action; to limit regressive, intrusive, maladaptive dependency; to reinforce autonomy; and to cultivate collaboration.

> **Key words:** abuse, autonomy, boundaries, countertransference enactment, dependency, emergencies, evocative memory, exploitation, frame, intersubjectivity, limit setting, object constancy, psychotherapy, safety, self-discipline, suicide, therapeutic contract

10

No-Shows, Late Arrivals, and Late Departures

Psychiatric emergency departments, many substance abuse counseling centers, and numerous neighborhood mental health centers welcome patients on a walk-in basis. In contrast, psychotherapy of virtually all types is conducted by appointment only. A scheduled appointment ensures that the therapist will be available, and that the patient will meet with the same therapist each time.

Patients' late arrivals, absences without notice ("no-shows"), or delays in leaving at the end of the appointment can be frustrating for the clinician. If these occurrences are explored tactfully and empathically, they may ultimately prove to be treasure troves of meaningful communication.

A LATE ARRIVAL

As a trainee, I looked forward to the sessions with my psychotherapy patients. About half an hour before a patient was scheduled to arrive, I would obsessively prepare the office for our upcoming meeting: moving the clock to an unobtrusive corner of the room, plumping the pillows on her chair, checking tissue availability. . . . I was ready to start the session about 15 minutes ahead of schedule.

After such preparation, I was painfully aware if my patient wasn't absolutely punctual. I'd repeatedly check the waiting room a minute after she was due to arrive, and if I didn't see her, my imagination would start to wander. Maybe my patient had experienced an extraordinary metamorphosis since our last meeting. Perhaps she had dyed her hair blond and grown 3 inches since our last visit. If an accelerated aging process had occurred over the last 7 days, she might be the older woman sitting in the corner knitting a sweater.

These creative fantasies were a bit bizarre, but in retrospect, I understand how they were protective. My odd musings helped me to wait and to contain my anticipation. If my patient were present, even disguised in a new form, I would have something else to do rather than to mark time forlornly near the secretary, peering at the clinic's entrance.

HOW TO REACT TO THE LATE-ARRIVING PATIENT

I imagined that my supervisors could transform a patient's late arrival into a therapeutic breakthrough. After listening to the patient's complaints about traffic on the way to the office, they would pounce on the issue: "So, it's difficult to come on time? What do you feel this means about the treatment?" In my fantasy, the patient wouldn't respond defensively, but would engage instead in a barrage of psychologically meaningful associations. Together, the two of them would rapidly come to a new and deeper understanding of her unconscious.

With experience and consultation, I've realized that my imagining is a bit fantastical, and my aspirations have become more humble and less dramatic. When I related my therapeutic expectations in response to a late arrival, my supervisors informed me that it is not useful to assign significant psychological meaning to a single event. Even when an unconscious drive is fueling the tardiness, direct and somewhat insensitive confrontations often lead to defensiveness and withdrawal rather than to increased insight. I stopped hoping for the psychological epiphany, and became more interested in how late arrivals might subtly affect the process of an ongoing treatment.

As a novice therapist, I was often overaccommodating when a patient was late. Although my intentions were good, extending the session to make up for the lost time had unforeseen clinical consequences.

EXAMPLE 10.1

The therapist is overaccommodating and extends the session to placate a late patient

SALLIE: (*rushing in 20 minutes late*) Dr. Bender, I got stuck in traffic. I couldn't call to tell you that I was going to be late because I didn't want to waste a moment. I'm so frustrated!

THERAPIST: I can understand that feeling. Why don't we go in and get started?

We walk together to the office.

SALLIE: So, I have so much to tell you. I've told you about my friend Gwen, who had been my most supportive buddy after the breakup with Charlie? Well, lately she's changed, and I have no idea why. She rarely calls me anymore, and when we do talk, she seems sort of distant. [*Sallie continues to talk about her concerns until 5 minutes before the end of the session.*]

THERAPIST: It seems that your relationship with Gwen has become more complicated. I hope we can continue to discuss it next week.

SALLIE: Dr. Bender, I need to talk to you more today. This situation with Gwen is difficult, but something just happened at home that is really horrible, I wanted to bring it up earlier, but I was scared to because I hate even thinking about it. Honestly, my problems with Gwen are stupid in comparison. Please, could we talk a little longer? It wasn't my fault that the traffic was so bad.

THERAPIST: [*I'm very curious and decide to extend the session.*] Okay, just this once. It's generally important to stick to our allotted appointment time, but we can take that up in a future visit. What is going on at home?

SALLIE: Well, I didn't really tell you much about this before, but my brother, Tom, is actually pretty sick. He has this problem with diarrhea.

It's sort of embarassing to talk about, but sometimes it gets so bad he has to go into the hospital. I think it is called ulcerative colitis or something like that. Anyway, when I was in high school, he had his first attack and he was in the hospital for weeks. He had to go to the bathroom about 30 times a day, and it was bloody too. My Dad would sleep at home with me, and my Mom slept at the hospital with Tom. I almost never saw her, but that was okay. I knew that Tom needed her more than I did.

What's strange is that sometimes he gets better, and then he's totally normal. For the last few years, he had been doing really well. But last night my parents called, and said that he had to go back to the hospital yesterday. It sounds like he's doing really bad again, and no one knows now long it will take for him to get better again. (*Sobs, and reaches for tissues.*)

THERAPIST: Oh, I can understand why this unexpected news was very upsetting.

1 Minute to Go before Session is Over

SALLIE: Right now, he is not allowed to eat, and he only gets food in his veins. My parents are both very upset, but my Mom is a total mess.

I asked her what I could do to help, and you know what she said? It's kinda strange.

THERAPIST: [*I can't resist.*] What did she say?

SALLIE: She said hearing about my courses, my economics courses, helps her feel a little better. She said it distracts her from the hospital and all that stuff. When she thinks about my future in business, it really makes her happy.

So there was no way that I could tell her that I hate my classes right now. They are SO boring, but I tried to sound really interested, because I didn't want to burden her more. (*Blows her nose.*)

THERAPIST: What a tough position to be in. Can you tell me more about how you experience this burden?

SALLIE: She thinks I like business as much as she does. I like it, I guess, but I don't love it. I think she would be bummed if she knew this.

The Hour is Up

THERAPIST: (*Nods, concerned look.*)

SALLIE: I just didn't want to talk to you about this before.

THERAPIST: [*I don't even begin to wrap up the session.*] What allowed you to bring it up with me today?

SALLIE: I don't know. Maybe the fact that he went back into the hospital and I needed to talk to somebody about it. But, part of me sort of hopes that if I don't talk about it, it might just go away.

THERAPIST: What does it feel like to talk about it with me?

SALLIE: Surprisingly okay. Maybe it took more energy to ignore it. I really appreciate you extending the hour for me, Dr. Bender. Gwen isn't there for me, but you certainly are!

The conversation continued for 15 minutes beyond the scheduled ending time. I miss my 10-minute break after Sallie's session and am late for my next patient.

Interestingly enough, patients who arrive late and patients who are reluctant to leave are often one and the same. Sallie illustrates the "hand-on-the-doorknob" phenomenon, sharing the session's most emotionally intense information at the end of the hour. Sometimes patients employ this tactic—often unconsciously—when they don't feel comfortable talking about a topic in detail. In Sallie's case, she may also be unconsciously trying to push the time limits of the session by ending with powerful material.

As Sallie is not acutely suicidal, it is not in her best interest to bend the treatment frame excessively, as I do in Example 10.1. An extension in even a single session may have a number of future ramifications: Sallie might continue to request prolonged sessions, and her motivation for arriving on time might diminish. Even though she might appreciate the extra time and attention, it may also feel confusing if I vary a session's length depending on its content. A 60-minute session could be regarded as an unexpected reward, while a shorter, 45-minute session could be viewed as a punishment.

If I prolong the session, it will be difficult to engage Sallie in an exploration of her end-of-the-hour actions. In contrast, if I end the session on time, Sallie will still be in touch with the feelings that fueled her request for an extended session. In a subsequent meeting, I can ask her how she experienced my limit setting and try to learn why it was difficult for her to talk about Tom's illness earlier in the meeting.

Example 10.2 illlustrates how I could hold firm to a treatment's boundaries in an empathic but resolute manner.

EXAMPLE 10.2

The therapist does not extend a session to accommodate a patient who was late

Five Minutes Left to the Session

SALLIE: Dr. Bender, I need to talk to you more today. This situation with Gwen is difficult, but something just happened at home that is really horrible. . . . Please, could we extend the session a little today?

THERAPIST: I would like to hear what you want to tell me, but we will need to stop on time. I would like to know what is on your mind, and then we can definitely continue to talk about it next week.

SALLIE: Next week seems so far away. The problem is that my brother Tom is in the hospital again. I don't remember if I told you, but he has this kind of rare chronic disease. He's been fine for years, but now he is having a relapse.

THERAPIST: Oh, I can understand that can be very upsetting. What kind of chronic illness does he have?

SALLIE: It's called ulcerative colitis. If he doesn't get better, he may need to have surgery. I just don't know what to do! (*Sniffles continue; reaches for a tissue and blows her nose.*)

THERAPIST: [*I refrain from asking exploratory questions such as "What allowed you to bring it up today?" or "What does it feel like to talk about it with me?" and I start to sum up instead.*] I can see this has been very painful and I hope we can talk about it in more detail next time. I know it may feel difficult to end our sessions once an issue like this comes up, but, unfortunately, we need to stop soon.

SALLIE: Oh, it just feels overwhelming. Dr. Bender, he is so sick. I need help dealing with this! Why won't you help me?

THERAPIST: (*gripping the chair*) [*metaphorically gripping the frame*] I feel stuck because I really do want to hear more about this, but unfortunately there isn't time to talk to you about it right now. Would it be helpful to schedule an extra session to talk more about this later in the week?

SALLIE: No. I don't have time. You can't talk now, even just 20 minutes more? (*A tear rolls down her cheek.*)

Sallie's Session Is Over

THERAPIST: I can see that the situation with your brother is so upsetting to you, and I understand that it was difficult for you even to let me know about it. Unfortunately, this session is ending at a really inopportune time. Why don't you take a moment to collect yourself and decide whether you want to meet later in the week with me so we can give it the time it deserves?

SALLIE: (*Nods, hiccups, doesn't move from her seat.*)

THERAPIST: (*Nods, and waits patiently.*)

SALLIE: (*Grabs a handful of tissues and stands up.*) It is so hard to talk about this, so I don't think I want to think about it again this week. Let's just meet next week as usual.

THERAPIST: Okay. That would be fine. I look forward to seeing you then.

SALLIE: Okay. (*Leaves.*)

In Example 10.2, I follow each empathic comment with a remark about the end of the session, and Sallie leaves the meeting within a couple minutes of the appropriate time. If she brings up emotionally intense material at the end of future sessions, we will try together to understand the meaning of this behavior.

EXAMPLE 10.3

When a patient repeatedly brings up emotionally loaded topics at the end of the session

One week after Sallie tells me about her brother's illness for the first time.

Five Minutes Before Sallie's Session Is Over

SALLIE: Enough about Gwen. I guess I didn't talk very much about my brother, Tom, today even though I planned to bring it up earlier this session. I need to tell you more about what is going on.

THERAPIST: (*Nods.*)

SALLIE: Dr. Bender, this week has really been the pits. I'm such a mess. Either I'm worried about Gwen or upset about Charlie, but it's all over if I even start thinking about Tom. I'm so worried about him.

THERAPIST: What are you most worried about?

SALLIE: I just feel so bad for him, but I get overwhelmed even thinking about it. I don't know why I talked about Gwen today instead of Tom.

THERAPIST: Do you have any understanding why you talked about Gwen instead?

SALLIE: I don't know. Maybe it's easier to talk about Gwen and distract myself from what is really bothering me.

THERAPIST: That could be so. Not many people recognize such possibilities. [*I recognize and support Sallie's psychological mindedness.*]

SALLIE: I wish we could keep talking about it now.

THERAPIST: It is a difficult situation. I can see this is such a sensitive topic, but by bringing it up at the end of the hour rather than earlier, we don't have the opportunity to talk about it together. Our time today is drawing to a close, but I hope we can continue learning about this.

SALLIE: Okay. (*Gets up to leave.*)

When I hold to the parameters of the session, Sallie is able to acknowledge how difficult it is for her to talk about her brother's illness. In a future session, she also might share how she felt when I didn't extend the session in response to her request.

REPEATED LATE ARRIVALS

For some patients, arriving late to therapy, canceling at the last minute, or not showing up at all may become a recurrent problem. Because this behavior is a detriment to the therapy, it deserves some special attention.

Before I broach this topic with a patient, I try to distinguish whether the frequent late arrivals are due to obstructions or resistances to the therapy. Obstructions are factors out of a patient's control and often unpredictable (such as blizzards, floods, lack of transportation, or an illness in the patient or in the patient's family). Resistances to therapy refer to anything that interferes with the progress of therapy over which the patient has some influence (missing the bus, cancelling because of a minor ailment or an optional scheduling conflict). Some events are more difficult to label as obvious obstructions or resistances (such as an unanticipated change in the patient's schedule that interferes with the therapy appointment), and I reserve judgment for these events until more information is available.

Whether or not the recurrent lateness is due to a resistance or to an obstruction, or a combination of the two, a discussion about lateness should be approached with empathy and curiosity. Timing is also important. As a beginning resident, I'd be so eager to broach the topic, that I'd open a session by asking a patient about her tardiness. Not surprisingly, the discussion was rarely fruitful. It took me a while to learn that the best time to explore a late arrival or a missed session is not necessarily the first available second in the next scheduled meeting. Instead, I've learned to wait for a cue, that is, some comment by the patient about time, appointments, or people in her life who are late. Then I'll ask the question I've been harboring: "I've noticed that sometimes you have been coming to the therapy session about 15 minutes late. Any thoughts about what might make it hard to come on time for some sessions?"

At the beginning of Example 10.4, Sallie Gane refuses to admit that her recurrent late arrivals have any underlying meaning, but as our meeting continues, she is increasingly able to discuss the emotional significance of her actions.

EXAMPLE 10.4

Discussing repeated late attendance in a therapeutic manner

Sallie came to the session 20 minutes late today. She was also 10–15 minutes late for the three sessions before this one.

When the session has only 10 minutes remaining, she starts to talk faster.

SALLIE: You won't believe the latest incident with Gwen. Last night, she wanted to go to this foreign movie, and when I said I'd rather see the latest release for the school's Alfred Hitchcock revival, she hung up on me. This was one of the few times I even disagreed with her plans a little bit, and she responded by shutting me out! My night was ruined. I don't know what I did wrong, or what made her so mad. Maybe I am just a social failure.

THERAPIST: Gwen wasn't open to any discussion about the evening's activities?

SALLIE: That's right, but I should have just gone to the foreign flick. The last time Gwen and I got in a tiff like this I didn't want to spend an afternoon shopping in the city with her, because I had a paper due. We didn't talk for a few weeks. It felt like forever. I can't afford to lose her now, because I need all the support I can get, especially with Tom being sick.

THERAPIST: It's difficult when a friendship that means so much is unable to sustain little disagreements.

SALLIE: It really is. Maybe I need some more friends so I don't have to depend on Gwen so much, but I have trouble making new friends. I get shy.

THERAPIST: It's important to talk about this, but we don't have the time today to talk about it in the detail it deserves. We only have a couple of minutes left.

SALLIE: Yeah, I wish I had more time.

THERAPIST: [*I grab the opportunity to talk about Sallie's recurrent lateness.*] Any idea of what might be making it hard to come on time?

SALLIE: I don't know. . . . It's not easy to talk about this stuff every week, you know.

THERAPIST: (*Nods encouragingly.*)

SALLIE: Can I tell you just one more thing? It'll just take a minute.

THERAPIST: We do need to stop, but I hope we can continue this discussion in the future. Perhaps the fact that it's not easy to talk about these painful topics has some influence on your lateness. It can be useful to try to understand it together, and maybe we can start to puzzle it out at our next meeting.

Sallie comes to the next session 15 minutes late.

SALLIE: Well, a lot has happened with Gwen since our last meeting.

THERAPIST: (*Nods encouragingly.*)

SALLIE: Well, like I expected, we didn't talk all week because I didn't go with her to that stupid movie. Then, she called yesterday and pretended nothing had ever happened. She invited me to a dorm barbeque, and we had a great time. I guess everything is normal between us again.

THERAPIST: How do you feel now that the relationship is back to baseline?

SALLIE: I'm so relieved. I don't know what I would do without Gwen. Other than you, she is my number one support in college. No offense, but talking to you once a week isn't enough. Gwen's an important part of my life here.

THERAPIST: No offense taken. I agree with you that it is really important for you to have close friends. How did you feel when Gwen pretended that your argument had never happened?

SALLIE: I felt so lucky. I would hate to talk to her about our disagreement.

THERAPIST: What would you hate about it?

SALLIE: I'd be scared that I might say something wrong, and she'd stop talking to me again. I can't afford to jeopardize my friendship with Gwen in any way.

THERAPIST: The friendship with Gwen is so important to you, but it also feels rather fragile?

SALLIE: You bet. I've seen her drop other friends in an instant. She collects friends, and then every so often she cleans house and discards the "uninteresting" ones. Sometimes she makes me feel like the best friend she has ever had, but she also has a definite mean streak.

   The difference between us is that she can make a new friend in 5 minutes, but I'm more shy. I need her more than she needs me.

THERAPIST: It's hard.

SALLIE: Yeah, I hate talking openly about feelings.

THERAPIST: We spoke a little last week about what might be making it difficult to come to sessions on time, and I'm wondering if it could be related to the fact that you hate talking openly about feelings. What do you think?

SALLIE: No, I don't think it relates at all. Do you?

THERAPIST: Maybe. I had some thoughts about it. Let me know how they sound to you. Maybe if you had some feelings that were hard to express directly to me, it might be more difficult to come on time.

SALLIE: What do you mean?

THERAPIST: Well, with Gwen, you have been concerned that more direct communication would lead to difficulties within the friendship. It makes sense that you might have mixed feelings within any relationship, and avoiding the issue is one way to cope with these feelings.

Coming late to therapy could be one way to protect yourself from talking about any mixed feelings you might have about our work. [*I feel proud to unveil my interpretation.*]

SALLIE: I don't have any mixed feelings about you.

THERAPIST: You don't? [*My interpretation didn't work? I had been perfecting it all week.*]

SALLIE: No, I don't. Dr. Bender, you are so important to me. I really treasure our sessions. I don't really understand what you are getting at.

THERAPIST: None of what I said fits with your experience? [*It's hard to give up my interpretation that I am so proud of, but it's becoming clear that, at this point in the treatment, Sallie isn't able to talk about our relationship so openly.*]

SALLIE: No, it just makes me nervous, that's all. I don't think you are right. If I'm late it is because of traffic, that's all.

Sallie is beginning to sound annoyed. I try to reinforce our therapeutic alliance.

THERAPIST: I'm glad you correct me so I can try to understand the situation better.

I've been asking about your lateness for the sake of the therapeutic process. When the session starts late, it reduces the time we have to work together.

SALLIE: I guess it does, but traffic is traffic, that's all.

THERAPIST: (*Nods, remains quiet to see what Sallie talks about next.*)

SALLIE: Well, it's hard to come here and talk about all this stuff, even though I generally feel better when I leave.

THERAPIST: Can you pinpoint what is hard about it?

SALLIE: Well, I sometimes get a little worried about what you think of me. I don't want you thinking that I am some kind of whiner who can't keep friends.

THERAPIST: Is that what you imagine that I think? (*curiously; nonconfrontational tone*)

SALLIE: I don't know. I just worry that one day you might get so sick of hearing what I have to say that you tell me to shut up. I talk about the same stuff every week, and even though I know that we are making progress, I figure you must feel sort of frustrated.

THERAPIST: Have I seemed frustrated to you?

SALLIE: No, you haven't at all, but maybe you are the type of person who is really patient for a long time but then erupts without warning.

THERAPIST: It is hard to trust that I won't become unpredictable and mean, sort of like Gwen?

SALLIE: I hadn't really thought about that, but I guess that is true.

THERAPIST: I can understand why this could hold you back. Can you tell me more?

SALLIE: What if I do say something offensive, and you are upset with me?

THERAPIST: Upset in what way?

SALLIE: Mad, angry, frustrated, bored . . . I don't know. I don't want to mess up this therapy. It's helping me.

THERAPIST: Actually, it is very useful to discuss this together in order to learn more about the feelings involved. Let's imagine for the sake of the therapy that I might feel some of the feelings you listed. What would that be like for you?

SALLIE: Oh, I'd be terrified.

THERAPIST: Can you tell me why?

SALLIE: Because the relationship would be over. . . .

THERAPIST: How so?

SALLIE: Well, you probably wouldn't want to work with me anymore.

THERAPIST: Why not?

SALLIE: Because you'd be pissed.

THERAPIST: I can see why this is so scary. There is a feeling that if there is any type of misunderstanding or disagreement between us, the therapy would be over.

SALLIE: Yes. I would be very worried if I made you angry.

THERAPIST: What would you imagine would happen?

SALLIE: I don't know. I guess I'd feel really uncomfortable talking to you.

THERAPIST: Tell me if this sounds possible to you. You might expect that our relationship would be similar to your friendship with Gwen. It wouldn't be resilient, so it couldn't easily sustain a misunderstanding.

SALLIE: Yes, actually that does sound right.

THERAPIST: Do you think that being late might be protective in some way?

SALLIE: Well, I have less opportunity to be annoying if I'm not here the whole time. Even if you are a little annoyed at me for being late, I know I can be on really good behavior for 30 minutes.

THERAPIST: So, by being late, you are trying to protect our relationship?

SALLIE: I know it sounds stupid, but maybe I am.

THERAPIST: I don't think it sounds stupid at all. I am glad we can talk openly about it, and we might understand it even better together over time.

Many patients, especially those new to psychotherapy, are similar to Sallie at the onset of Example 10.4. They may have trouble talking openly about their recurrent late arrivals, and the therapist must facilitate the discussion slowly and sensitively.

Midway into Example 10.4, I illustrate what can happen if the therapist pursues a more aggressive approach. I take control of the session's content when I introduce my carefully concocted interpretation: "Coming late to therapy could be one way to protect yourself from talking about any mixed feelings you might have about our work." Sallie balks and is unable to process my comment in any meaningful way. I realize that the interpretation was premature when it doesn't facilitate a more open and honest discussion, and Sallie adamantly repeats that her recurrent late arrivals are meaningless.

The conversation does progress in the second half of the example as Sallie morphs into a patient with more psychological insight, and I evolve into a therapist with more experience. I try to clarify Sallie's concerns ("It is hard to trust that I won't become unpredictable and mean, sort of like Gwen?") instead of presenting sweeping interpretations. I learn about Sallie's fear that she may not maintain appropriate behavior if she comes to her session on time, a very different explanation for her recurrent tardiness than the interpretation I had offered earlier.

Sallie's late arrivals may have many meanings. At this time, Sallie believes it is only an attempt to avoid confrontation, but it may also be her method of expressing hostility and resentment. Even if this conjecture is valid, Sallie appears far from ready to recognize her own animosity. It is not the right time to talk to her about this second possibility, so I think about it silently.

As Sallie's therapist, I also start to wonder why Sallie has trouble making new friends, and why she is so attached to Gwen even though Gwen treats her poorly. Early in treatment, I can only hypothesize some explanations. Maybe Sallie perceives Gwen as irreplaceable because Gwen is somehow symbolically tied to someone in Sallie's life who does have a unique and vital role, such as her mother, father, or brother. We'll learn more about this as the therapy continues.

RECURRENT CANCELLATIONS OR NO-SHOWS

While late arrivals can be annoying, at least the patient shows up. As a trainee, I found cancellations or no-shows the most aggravating, mainly because I would bend over backward to try to accommodate my patient when rescheduling.

The typical scenario would unfold as follows. My patient would miss her scheduled appointment by cancelling or not showing up. Then, she'd call shortly afterward to apologize and to attempt to reschedule within the next few days. I'd feel concerned and, in order to meet as soon as possible, I would reschedule the patient in the evening or early in the morning. If I was lucky, the patient would show for this session, but sometimes the pattern would continue, and my resentment would escalate exponentially.

With experience, I've learned a different strategy that also protects my time. I use the patient's request to reschedule as a moment to reassert the frame. Unless there is a compelling emergency, I set the next appointment at our regularly scheduled time during the following week.

The situation is more tricky if the no-shows become a chronic problem.

EXAMPLE 10.5

Responding to a patient who recurrently misses her appointments

Sallie has just finished the consultation process, but then misses her first scheduled therapy session and does not call to cancel.

I call her and leave the following message, hoping to demonstrate interest.

"Hello, this is Suzanne Bender, calling for Sallie Gane. After I did not see you at our meeting today, I wondered if you were interested in rescheduling. If so, please leave me a message with some times that I could reach you."

Sallie calls back 2 days later and leaves the following message.

"Oh, Dr. Bender, I got your message. I am very sorry I missed our appointment. I had a final at school the morning of our meeting, and I just completely forgot about our session. I still am very interested in therapy. Please call me so we can reschedule."

I call Sallie back, and after we reschedule I mention my cancellation policy. I explain that unless there are extenuating circumstances, I will charge her for future appointments unless she calls to cancel at least 48 hours in advance.

She misses her next appointment without calling to cancel.

A second missed appointment is less likely to be due to chance alone. Unless I am worried that Sallie may be in some danger, I don't immediately call her after the second no-show.

For Sallie, the process of psychotherapy may feel comforting, revealing, and frightening at the same time. In response, she may feel simultaneously pulled toward and pushed away from treatment. If I call her back immediately after each missed session, she may react in an avoidant manner. If I wait before contacting her, she may feel less external pressure to continue therapy and may be able to experience both sides of her ambivalence. Then, if she decides to pursue treatment, it will be an independent decision, fueled by her desire for emotional relief.

After Sallie's second no-show, I'll wait a few days to a week before calling her.

If I'm unable to contact her directly, my second phone message may be similar to the first with the addendum: "If I do not hear from you, I shall assume you are not interested in meeting at this time, and I shall close your file. If an emergency arises, please contact your nearest emergency room."

At the end of the month, I will send Sallie a bill, including a charge for the second meeting that she missed.

With two cancellations in a row, Sallie's ambivalence about psychotherapy is tilting toward aversion and avoidance. Unless the therapy can help her to talk openly about her recurrent no-shows, her resistance will continue unabated. If she contacts me in the future, I will make sure that we talk about the two no-shows shortly after she returns.

Sallie calls back a few weeks after her second missed appointment and my second phone response.

SALLIE: Dr. Bender, I am so sorry I missed my last appointment. But now that school is out, I'd like to set up a time to meet. I have a lot to tell you.

THERAPIST: Okay. Unfortunately, the times I have available are relatively limited right now.

SALLIE: That's okay. I have a very flexible schedule during my break. Just name the time.

THERAPIST: How is Thursday at 11:00? [*I choose a time to meet that is very convenient for me. In case Sallie doesn't show up, I will go to an early lunch.*]

SALLIE: Great! Perfect! I'll see you then. Thank you so much.

THERAPIST: If for any reason, you find that you will be unable to make the appointment, please call to cancel, preferably 48 hours in advance.

Thursday arrives. Five minutes after 11:00, I check my voice mail. Sallie had left a message at 11:00 that she was unable to find a parking place and would be late for our appointment.

At 20 minutes after the hour, Sallie rushes into the clinic, apologizing profusely.

SALLIE: Dr. Bender, it is so good to finally see you again. I am sorry I am late. I hope you got my message. I guess I'll have to talk fast. Recently, I have been really depressed.

THERAPIST: How would you describe the depressed feeling?

For the next 10 minutes, I focus on Sallie's main concern and assess whether she is at any risk.

THERAPIST: With all this pain and turmoil, perhaps part of you didn't want to come to our sessions to talk about it even though another part of you wanted some help and comfort.

SALLIE: I don't know. Well, I guess I have felt pulled both ways.

THERAPIST: That is how it is with a lot of people. If you decide you want to look into it more, we can keep meeting and learn what will be best for you in your situation. Also, if you want to stop treatment now because it doesn't feel like the right time to be in therapy, that is okay too.

If Sallie continues to miss sessions after this discussion, she may be too ambivalent about therapy to continue at this time. Even if she repeatedly states that she is interested in treatment, she is "voting with her feet." I would follow up with a letter (see Figure 10.1).

My letter purposely does not guarantee future treatment. If Sallie decides to stop treatment for the time being and then contacts me months later, ready to start, I will agree initially to meet for only one consultation visit. After the single-session consultation, Sallie and I can discuss her treatment options: continuing with me if I have the time available, placing her name on my waiting list for my next open time slot if the need is not urgent, or finding a new therapist who can meet her current clinical needs.

CANCELLATION POLICIES

Cancellation policies vary widely among therapists. Some therapists consider a patient's session a rented hour and require that the patient pay

---

[Use the clinic's letterhead.]

Date

Ms. Sallie Gane
1111 Central Street
Boston, MA 02114

Dear Ms. Gane:

I am writing to you because I'm unclear about your decision regarding future treatment since we last met on MM/DD/YY.

I don't, of course, have any way of knowing what's going on with you currently, but I hope things are better.

If you want to be in touch with me about future psychotherapy, I would be happy to meet with you to discuss your treatment needs. I wish you well.

Sincerely,

Suzanne Bender, MD

voice mail#

FIGURE 10.1. Letter inviting the patient to resume contact.

for a cancelled meeting if the therapist is not able to find someone else to fill the time. Some therapists, with more chutzpah than I, even require the patient to pay for sessions when the therapist is on vacation! Neither of these policies have ever felt quite right to me.

I tell patients about my cancellation policy during the consultation or after the patient has missed her first session. I require 48 hours notice for a cancelled session. I will charge for the missed hour if the cancellation occurs less than 48 hours before the session.

Of course, every rule has its exceptions. I don't charge for cancelled sessions until I've explained my policy to the patient, and I don't charge if the patient cannot come to her appointment due to extenuating circumstances such as a snowstorm or unexpected significant illness in the patient or a family member (in other words, an obstruction). A rare patient may take advantage of this flexibility and concoct incredible excuses for frequently missed sessions. In such a situation, I may start charging for all future missed sessions, after explaining to the patient that I am unwilling to save a session without payment. But this situation is extremely unusual. Usually, the cancellation policy protects the therapy. Once a patient realizes that she may be financially responsible for a missed session, I've been amazed at how quickly attendance rates improve.

With patients who are using their insurance to pay for treatment, cancellation policies are not as straightforward. Insurance policies don't reimburse clinicians if a patient doesn't show up. For a private practice, it may be possible to negotiate a payment agreement with my patient, so she will pay for abruptly cancelled sessions while the insurance will subsidize the sessions that do occur. (This agreement must comply with any restrictions outlined by the insurance carrier.) With a clinic practice, I may not have this luxury, but it is still useful to discuss the recurrent missed sessions. I'd remind the patient that the appointments that are not cancelled with adequate notice cannot be made available to patients who might benefit from them. Sometimes people who are neglectful of their own well-being (and their own psychotherapy) may act more responsibly when they realize that their behavior might deprive or harm others.

Some clinic treaters ask their patients to make a donation to a charity for every missed session. If the patient is able and willing, this policy can act as an informal cancellation agreement. Since the patient has only a moral obligation to make the donation, the policy lacks any bite behind its bark.

If after lengthy discussions a clinic patient continues to abuse the privilege of a weekly reserved hour, I might taper her access to my services. Possibly with sessions on alternate weeks, she might be able to come more regularly. If the no-shows continue unabated, I might talk to the patient about deferring further treatment until she can demonstrate that she is able to proceed on a regular basis. In such a situation, I would also remind her of the availability of emergency services should the need arise.

THE THERAPIST IS LATE TO A SESSION

When the therapist is late to a session, a different set of dynamics come into play.

EXAMPLE 10.6

The therapist is late to the session

On the way to the clinic to see Sallie at 2:00 P.M., I realize that I left my wallet sitting on the table in the cafeteria. I rush back, retrieve the wallet, and then run to the clinic. I am 10 minutes late. It is the first time I have been late for a session since I have started working with Sallie.

THERAPIST: (*a bit breathless from running to the clinic*) Please come on in.

SALLIE: (*Looks quizzically at me.*) So, I have a lot to tell you about Gwen.

THERAPIST: Yes. I'm sorry to have kept you waiting.

SALLIE: Oh, I knew something unusual must have come up. It's okay. I'm not too picky about starting on time.

THERAPIST: If you have any feelings about the fact I was late, please feel free to share them with me.

SALLIE: Nah, the stuff with Gwen is much more pressing.

THERAPIST: Are you able to stay an extra 10 minutes so we can make up the time?

SALLIE: Sure, that would be great. [*Proceeds to talk about Gwen*]

Ten Minutes Later

SALLIE: Umm, I did have this weird thought that crossed my mind when you were late.

THERAPIST: I am glad you bring it up. What was it?

SALLIE: Well, I know this sounds paranoid, but I heard about a really bad car accident on the radio on the way here, and I was worried that maybe you were in it. Where were you anyway?

THERAPIST: You were worried that I was hurt?

SALLIE: Yeah, I felt a little scared.

THERAPIST: Can you tell me what you were scared of?

SALLIE: Umm, well, what if you were badly hurt? I don't want anything bad to happen to you. If you were late all the time, I wouldn't have been so worried. But you have never been late before so I got sort of freaked out.

THERAPIST: It sounds like it was somewhat frightening.

SALLIE: I guess it was.

THERAPIST: For the sake of our work together, can you tell me more about what you imagined? What did you imagine had happened to me in the car accident?

SALLIE: I don't know. That feels like a weird question. I think I'm just wired this way. I usually get worried when people are late for a meeting. Gwen might be an exception, though. She's late all the time and I don't ever worry about her. Maybe I don't care about her in the same way. [*continues to talk about her feelings about people being late*]

While some patients are unable to talk openly about a therapist's late arrival (Sallie at the beginning of Example 10.6), others will use the event to further the therapy (Sallie at the end of Example 10.6).

Over time, it may become clear that Sallie may have a barrage of feelings about my late arrival. While she may feel concerned and worried up front, other feelings, including anger or disappointment about the lost time, may surface in the future.

If I am late for a session, I will extend the meeting to make up for lost time. Some very traditional therapists will end the session on time believing it is better to maintain a strict treatment frame and let the patient express how it feels to pay for a full hour but only receive a portion of it. We believe it is respectful and fair to extend the hour if other patients are not adversely affected.

Now and then, I'll tell the patient some details about my tardiness. If I arrive at the office covered in grease after changing a flat tire, it would be absurd to ignore the obvious and pretend nothing unusual had happened. Early on, I was at risk for sharing too much information ("My tire was acting strange all week, and I should have taken the subway. It blew three blocks from the office"), but all the patient really needs to know is the bare details ("I had to change my tire on the way to the office").

Some patients may also become overwhelmingly anxious if I'm late and may imagine that something terrible has happened in my life. In this type of situation, providing some information about my situation will alleviate the patient's anxiety and will facilitate a discussion of her emotional reaction.

It is especially meaningful if a therapist repeatedly breaks the frame with recurrent late arrivals. If such a sequence occurs, one's first reaction may be self-critical, but this response is actually the least helpful to the therapy. To help the treatment progress, it is more useful to give oneself credit for noticing the pattern of behavior and then schedule a discussion with a trusted supervisor in order to understand what the actions might signify. Just as in the case of the patient, once the underlying dilemma fueling the repeated tardiness is verbalized and understood (in this case, in supervision), it should become easier to be on time and less necessary to act in response to the feelings.

No-shows, late arrivals, and late departures are all actions relevant to the therapy whether they are produced by the patient or by the therapist. By translating the meaning of relevant actions into words, the therapist and patient gain greater understanding of the process and of themselves.

Key words: ambivalence, avoidant behavior, counterresistance, duration of sessions, intersubjectivity, obstruction, psychotherapy, psychotherapeutic contract, psychotherapeutic frame, resistance

11

Confidentiality and Its Limits

Your patient must be able to rely on confidentiality to make the highly personal and often exquisitely sensitive disclosures that are essential in psychotherapy. However, your patient should know that if she is at clear risk of harming herself or others, your first obligation is to protect. Occasionally, you may need to break confidentiality to ensure safety.

PROTECTING PATIENT INFORMATION

As a therapist, I am the antithesis of a traditional storyteller. I am a story holder, privy to the details of my patients' lives, their most private attitudes, wishes, and disappointments. To protect my patients, I am bound to a code of silence (or confidentiality, as it is called in professional circles); if I share information about a patient, it is only under specific and controlled conditions.

When I started training, it wasn't easy to adapt to the rules of my new profession. Emotionally laden information is inherently interesting, and part of me wanted to describe my patients' stories with my family and friends. During social gatherings, it was frustrating to refer to my work in vague technical terms as I listened to my nontherapist friends eagerly share the concrete details of their days.

In retrospect, I understand why it was so difficult to maintain confidentiality when I started this work. I craved emotional support after listening to my patients' suffering. I needed to debrief, but I wasn't sure whom I could tell.

I would have welcomed a "novice therapist information packet" that outlined the basics of confidentiality. Neophyte therapists need to know how to process their experience while simultaneously protecting a patient's privacy. This chapter attempts to satisfy that need.

TELLING THE SUPERVISOR

As my professional contacts increased, it became much easier to maintain my patients' confidentiality during conversations with my friends and family.

As a part of my training, I was required to review the details of my patients' treatments with three or four instructors each week. My assigned supervisors, all experienced psychotherapists, provided crucial guidance and support for my work. As integral members of the treatment team, they also bore some clinical responsibility and authority for a patient's therapy. With their help, I was able to develop an effective treatment strategy for each patient. Disclosure to a supervisor is allowed by law in most jurisdictions, but these specialized practitioners are also ethically and legally bound to keep all clinical information secure.

My supervisors became my trusted teachers and mentors. Our weekly meetings provided an approved professional structure in which I could talk openly about my concerns. With their help, I found it much easier to tolerate my patients' distress and to maintain clinical confidentiality.

As part of the informed consent requirement, patients who are under the care of a trainee need to be told that a supervisor is involved, from the diagnostic consultation to the therapy that might follow. (For further information on how to discuss a supervisor's involvement, please see Chapter 3.)

EXAMPLE 11.1

The therapist-in-training informs the patient that a supervisor will advise and guide the therapist

About halfway through our first session, Sallie and I decide on a future meeting time, and I tell her about my supervision.

THERAPIST: Before we talk a bit more about Charlie, I wanted to take a moment to tell you about my supervision.

As you know, this is a teaching hospital. One of the advantages of receiving your care here is that trainees, like me, receive advice regularly from experienced fully trained clinicians. To obtain that guidance, I'll have to give my supervisor information about you. I wanted to make sure to tell you this early in case you have any questions about it.

SALLIE: I don't know. I don't really want anyone else to know what we talk about.

THERAPIST: Can you tell me more what you are concerned about?

SALLIE: What will your teachers think of me? I don't want anyone else to know my business.

THERAPIST: I understand your wish for privacy. By law, my supervisor is required to keep the information that I share with him completely confidential.

It's important that you know that my supervisors are available for your benefit, not just mine. With their help, I will be able to provide you with the most comprehensive treatment.

I still seek clinical advice from my supervisors intermittently, even though I've been out of training for a number of years. This process is known as a consultation, and it's a tool even experienced clinicians use to ensure the quality of the care they're providing. Consultants are often selected among highly respected clinicians in the local mental health community. They usually charge a fee for their services. Unlike supervision during training, the consultant does not have any clinical authority or responsibility concerning the case.

During a consultation, I do not disclose my patient's identity. Unless there is a chance that the consultant will recognize the patient from the material presented, I do not need to obtain a patient's informed consent for the meeting.

TELLING OTHER CLINICIANS

There are some instances in which I disclose information to my patients' other health care providers. In general, all clinicians treating a patient, such as her internist, gynecologist, psychotherapist, or others, have the right to communicate with each other about a patient's treatment. Because psychotherapy is an especially private venture, it's best if the patient provides permission for these discussions with a verbal or, best of all, a written release of information. During discussions with other care providers, I use discretion and reveal only what is necessary for optimal medical care. I don't share irrelevant clinical details that may be potentially embarrassing to the patient.

TELLING A CONFERENCE

During my residency, my colleagues and I were often asked to summarize a patient's treatment for a clinical conference. Starting out, I felt very unsure about how to prepare for the conference but simultaneously protect the patient's privacy. To treat a patient with the same deference and respect she would receive during a session, we think that it makes the most sense for a patient to know if her clinical story is going to be presented at a formal conference. Here is one way that her informed consent could be obtained.

EXAMPLE 11.2

The therapist requests permission to consult a group of clinicians at a case conference

THERAPIST: I've been offered an opportunity to consult a group of psychotherapists at a conference. With your permission, I'd like to ask for their advice about your treatment.

SALLIE: Tell them about me?

THERAPIST: Yes, but without revealing your identity. I wouldn't tell them your name or the names of any of the people you have mentioned. Also I'd change a few facts that aren't essential to make it even less likely that you could be recognized.

SALLIE: I don't know. They might think my problems are stupid.

THERAPIST: That sounds like what you feel about your problems sometimes.
The people who will attend the conference will all be professionals. They'll respect your courage as I have. They will view the problems you and I are facing as just that: problems to be solved.

SALLIE: I'm not sure.

THERAPIST: You can think about it, and let's keep discussing it. We don't have to decide for a couple of weeks.

SALLIE: Will you be mad at me if I don't agree to it?

THERAPIST: No, I wouldn't be a bit mad, and we would continue working together as we have, but maybe we can learn a little more about that concern. How does it feel for me to request this of you?

In both oral and written presentations, I would mask my patient's identity by referring to her and to important people in her life by a pseudonym or an initial. For example, Sallie might be referred to as "X," and Gwen might be referred to as "Y." Even without a name, it's possible that a clinician at the conference might identify the patient by the details in the handout. For that reason, I will disguise the information further by altering facts that are not essential and by generalizing where possible. To avoid public dissemination of the handout's contents, I will collect all copies at the end of conference. I might keep one copy of my written presentation for my records, but I'll shred the rest of the papers after the meeting.

TELLING COLLEAGUES: WHERE AND WHEN

Sharing psychotherapy tips and discussing cases with my colleagues continue to be a mainstay of my professional development. With experience, though, I've become more stringent about when and where these discussions take place.

As an eager beginner, I'd try to avoid talking about patients in any open place where others could easily overhear, but I would have to reprimand myself often. I'd be at lunch in an open public area with one of my fellow residents and we would naturally fall into a discussion of our week's work. Occasionally, we'd catch ourselves spouting too much information midway into the conversation. Judging by my experience and observations of others, I can predict that many beginners will mention something about their patients in a public place early in training. Our hope is that by outlining the risks openly, the readers of this book will avoid these errors of confidentiality, both for the sake of their patients' privacy and their own medicolegal security.

I had been a psychiatric resident just a few weeks when a colleague of mine starting talking about his new psychotherapy patient while we rode on the subway. Even though he didn't mention the patient's name, he did share a number of identifying features of the patient as well as confidential information from the psychotherapy hour. I had an unusual visceral reaction, a mixture of interest and nausea.

Nowadays, I use this physical symptom as a personal cue. It means that I (or the person I am talking with) need to be more vigilant about confidentiality. While my method of visceral introspection may seem unusual, this sort of self-knowledge (autognosis) can be highly useful in life in general and in psychotherapy in particular.

Subways aren't the only common area of risk. Clinic waiting areas where colleagues converge to wait for upcoming patients can be prime places to overhear information that should stay behind closed doors.

Social gatherings, especially if a therapist's tongue is loosened with some alcohol, are also potential traps.

With experience, I've learned to avoid discussing case vignettes, even if I think I have sufficiently disguised a patient's identity, in heavily populated open spaces—or in closed public spaces like elevators. Even if it's unlikely that anyone overhearing the conversation might know my patient, open discussions aren't respectful of patients in general and reflect poorly on our profession.

If I could "do over" the subway incident, I would have exited the conversation the minute it felt inappropriate. When the topic became unsuitable for public consumption, a simple, "I don't think we should discuss this here. Let's talk about it later in a more private place" would have sufficed.

It is safest to relegate all discussions of patient information to private enclosed areas, such as an office. A phone conversation that cannot be overheard is also acceptable. It's worth avoiding cell phones as much as possible because others could theoretically intercept your conversation. Circumstances and opinions vary about the security of e-mail.

Rules, rules, and more rules. I imagine at least some readers believe we are proposing an overprotective approach to treatment. It's true that our rules may be more strict than those of other health care providers, but our work is often more sensitive. In some ways, a therapist's attention to confidentiality is akin to that of a community religious leader. All confidential information must be carefully cherished and protected.

Because of the careful attention we pay to confidentiality, practicing psychotherapy 40-50 hours a week and not being able to talk openly about work can be a pretty lonely experience. For this reason, many therapists mix teaching or writing with clinical practice. In public, one can talk freely about a class, paper, or book that is in progress in contrast to the more guarded approach appropriate for psychotherapeutic material.

WHAT SHOULD YOU WRITE IN YOUR NOTES?

In both my private and hospital clinic practices, I keep two sets of records for each patient. The offical psychiatric record of each patient at both sites includes a detailed write-up of the first consultation visit (chief complaint, past psychiatric and medical history, medications, etc.), a risk assessment for suicidality, and an outline of the treatment plan. For each followup visit, I record a short note that documents a patient's pertinent medical and safety information. I am very cautious about what I write in the notes that become part of the patient's medical record as this chart may be reviewed by other physicians or by insurance companies in the future. (See Figure 11.1 for a record of Sallie's psychotherapy session.)

For each psychotherapy patient, I also keep a second shadow file that includes more detailed notes reviewing my patients' more personal concerns. These process notes are for my personal use only, and I keep them in a protected area, separate from the official medical record. They may include details of each psychotherapy meeting in an "I said, she said" format, along with nonverbal communications and any questions and concerns I might think of during and after a patient's session. I don't include the patient's name on these notes, although it is safe to include a

---

Patient's name   Sallie Gane

Date 3/16/01   **Time of day** 11:30 A.M.

Duration of the session (50' psychotherapy)

Assessment of suicidality (SI) if appropriate
Occasional thoughts of death, but no wishes, intentions, plans, or actions. Good plans for immediate future.

Assessment of homicidality (HI) if appropriate
No history of violence. No intentions, plans, or actions.

Current medications
None

Any medication changes
N/A

Any change of symptoms related to medications
N/A

Adverse side effects
N/A

Return to clinic (RTC) date
3/23/01

Supervisor
Edward Messner, MD

Diagnosis
296.21

Treatment goals
1. Recovery from depression
2. Diminish rejection sensitivity

An overview of the issues being discussed (e.g., "family issues discussed")
Breakup with boyfriend. Conflicts with female friend.

FIGURE 11.1. Information included in a clinical psychotherapy note that will become part of the medical record.

coded designation on the papers, such as the patient's initials. (For more information on how to write process notes, see chapter 6.)

Each state has its own laws regarding a psychotherapist's obligation to document information. Our recommendations are based on our experience with Massachusetts law, so it might be worthwhile to understand your state's specific guidelines as well.

The two-note standard described herein complies with the Health Insurance Portability and Accountability Act (HIPAA), which will require a new standard of psychotherapy documentation on a national basis starting in 2003. These new regulations legally differentiate between medical record notes and psychotherapy process notes. The medical record should document medication prescription and monitoring, counseling session start and stop times, the modalities and frequencies of treatment, results of clinical tests, and any summary of the following items: diagnosis, functional status, the treatment plan, symptoms, prognosis, and progress. A separate file, such as process notes, is allowed, and described as a record or analysis of the conversations during a counseling session. The HIPAA maintains that these separate notes are only for the therapist's own use, and can be protected from others, including the patient, payer, other MD's, and so on.

While process notes are intended only for my personal use, it is currently impossible to guarantee that no one else will ever read them. For example, if my process notes are specifically subpoenaed by a court, I might be legally obligated to share the material. (Currently, legal obligations differ depending on the jurisdiction.) Because the future is unpredictable, I write all notes with the knowledge that someone else may read them someday. I avoid writing anything in any record that could be misunderstood about my own countertransference reaction toward the patient (disparaging, angry, or sexual feelings toward a patient, for example). These feelings deserve processing in supervision or in the clinician's own therapy, but documentation is risky. In case my notes were ever subpoenaed, a countertransference feeling or fantasy could be easily misconstrued by those in the judicial system, and might even be used as incriminating evidence. In the courts, there is a danger that a documented thought might carry as much weight as a corresponding action.

THE PATIENT WANTS TO SEE
HER OWN PSYCHOTHERAPY RECORD

Now and then, one of my patients becomes intensely interested in reviewing her own psychotherapy medical record. Example 11.3 illustrates how I might react to such a request from Sallie.

EXAMPLE 11.3

The therapist tries to learn the meaning behind the patient's request to see her own psychotherapy records

SALLIE: Dr. Bender, I was thinking after our last meeting that I would like to review the record of our sessions.

THERAPIST: Could you tell me what you are interested in reviewing?

SALLIE: Nothing really. I would just like to see what your notes say.

THERAPIST: I wonder what has sparked your interest.

SALLIE: Well, I just learned in psychology class that I have a legal right to review my own records. It sounded kind of interesting. Could we do it during the next session?

THERAPIST: You do have a legal right to review the records, but I think it is important that we approach this question just like anything else in therapy. Rather than just acting quickly, we should try to understand your request in more detail together.

SALLIE: There's nothing to it. I am just curious.

THERAPIST: What are you curious about?

SALLIE: I don't know, but sometimes I do sort of wonder what you think of me. Maybe it's a little hard to trust your niceness. So, I'd just like to check out the record, okay? (*a little defensive*)

THERAPIST: Can you say more about what is hard to trust about my niceness?

SALLIE: I don't know. I'm just interested if what I see is really what I get, if you know what I mean.

THERAPIST: What do you mean? I want to make sure I understand. (*with an encouraging tone*)

SALLIE: I don't know. I just don't feel as comfortable talking to you lately.

THERAPIST: When did you start to feel less comfortable?

SALLIE: Umm, I don't know.

THERAPIST: (*Nods.*) [*hoping to facilitate Sallie's associations*]

SALLIE: You just seemed a little distracted last week.

THERAPIST: (*Nods, empathic look.*) Distracted? Can you say more?

SALLIE: Well, I just felt you weren't as interested as you usually are.

THERAPIST: Can you tell me any more details? Did I seem uninterested during the whole meeting or at certain specific points?

SALLIE: I think the whole meeting. I just wondered if you were thinking about something else. I didn't want to bring it up though. I know we all have some days that are better than others.

THERAPIST: [*I thought I had listened attentively last week, and I don't know what Sallie perceived. I avoid the urge to defend myself.*] Did I say or act in any way in particular that made you feel like I was thinking about something else?

SALLIE: No, I just felt it.

THERAPIST: Do you feel it now?

SALLIE: Maybe a little bit. . . .

THERAPIST: I am glad you could tell me about this, and I can imagine that it is upsetting to you. I am sorry I added to your discomfort last week and right now as well. Maybe together we can learn more about what it going on between us and what I am not understanding.

SALLIE: Maybe. (*Tears appear in her eyes unexpectedly and she changes the topic.*)

Whenever a patient requests a change in the treatment frame, I try to understand the meaning behind the request in more detail before jumping to action. In this example, Sallie focuses on seeing her record when she feels I am less engaged in her treatment. Jumping to examine the record with her would have overlooked the concern driving her request. Her interest in the record becomes less urgent and even unimportant as the interview delves into the underlying issue.

If Sallie still wanted to see her psychotherapy record after an extensive therapeutic exploration, she has the legal right to do so. This situation does underline why it is prudent to write one's records with the consideration that someone else may read them someday. I would share the medical record version of my notes, as the process notes are written only for my personal use.

When I share my notes with a patient, we'll look at it together so as to avoid any further misunderstandings and confusion. I consider the discussion as part of the therapy, and it is often very fruitful. Some patients may wish I had written less, while others may feel that I haven't written enough. Either reaction is invariably the beginning of an interesting interchange.

My most challenging experience involving a medical record review request occurred when a paranoid patient in his 50s with a diagnosis of depression with psychotic features decided he wanted to review his medical record midway through treatment. He had no insight that his paranoia was part of his psychiatric disorder, and he was convinced that he was constantly being monitored by a government agency. I had documented that his paranoia was part of his psychosis in notes of my ongoing assessment, and I was worried about how he might react when he read this in his record.

He insisted on examining my notes, and before proceeding we talked about the process at length. I asked him how he might feel if I had or had not documented the possibility of a psychotic process in my medical notes. To strengthen the therapeutic alliance while we reviewed the notes, I documented his reaction during the process as a medical record addendum. For instance, when he became upset reading about the possibility of a psychotic diagnosis, he dictated: "Rex [not his real name] does not agree with Dr. Bender's assessment that his symptoms may be consistent with a diagnosis of depression with psychotic features. He feels very confident that the unusual phenomena he experienced did happen to him." We agreed to disagree about the cause of his symptoms and to my surprise, the therapeutic alliance not only survived but thrived.

For a subset of patients, viewing the psychiatric record could lead to a decompensation or even to a suicide or to violence. It would be countertherapeutic for these individuals to see any part of their medical therapy record, and I have some legal recourse to protect them. A clinic's or an insurance company's attorney will have the latest information regarding one's legal obligation and rights in this situation. Currently, in Massachusetts, the therapist can provide a treatment summary to a patient if she believes that reviewing the complete record with the patient directly would be clinically contraindicated.

If a patient continues to request her entire record rather than a summary, a statute in Massachusetts (Massachusetts General Laws, chapter 112, section 12CC) as of the year 2000 does provide some recourse:

> If in the reasonable exercise of his professional judgment, the psychotherapist believes providing the entire record would adversely affect the patient's well-being, the psychotherapist shall make the entire record available to either the patient's attorney, with the patient's consent, or to such other psychotherapist as designated by the patient.

While there is no similar federal statute, it is worthwhile checking on the particulars of your state's law. Hospitals, professional associations, and clinics usually have attorneys available who specialize in these types of situations. Whenever I have any legal questions, I obtain expertise early on.

SOMEONE WANTS PERSONAL INFORMATION ABOUT YOUR PATIENT

In certain instances, I may be asked to divulge information about my patient to a stranger. Unless it is an emergency, as we will discuss later in this chapter, I am bound first and foremost to protect my patient's confidentiality.

EXAMPLE 11.4

The therapist protects the patient's confidentiality in response to an unexpected phone call

Therapist's Office Phone Rings

GWEN: Hello, hello? Is this Dr. Bender?

THERAPIST: This is Dr. Bender. Who is this?

GWEN: Hi, my name is Gwen. I am a good friend of Sallie Gane's. I know you're her therapist. I wanted to call you, because I am really worried about Sallie. She's been acting strange lately, sort of distant or withdrawn. I don't know if something is very wrong. I figured you would want to know since you are her doctor.

THERAPIST: I cannot confirm whether Sallie Gane is my patient. [*I know that Sallie is searching for other friends and is slowly withdrawing from Gwen.*]

GWEN: Oh, I know she sees you. I just wanted to check to see if she is okay. She has been acting so weird lately. I'm pretty worried about her, and I didn't know who else to call.

THERAPIST: If you want to provide information about someone, I am willing to listen, but I cannot disclose whether any person is actually my patient.

GWEN: Well, what if Sallie is suicidal or something? You would need to do something—right? I don't think she's in any immediate danger, but I don't want to make any mistakes. A cousin of mine had a friend who killed herself, and no one saw it coming. So I wanted to do the right thing here.

THERAPIST: What I can tell you is that if any one of my patients were at risk for harming herself, I would be obligated by law to protect her and let the appropriate people know about her condition.

GWEN: But you can't tell me about Sallie specifically?

THERAPIST: I can only share my general policy regarding patient safety.

GWEN: Could you at least tell me if you think she's going to be okay? I don't know if I'm overreacting, but I really am worried about her.

THERAPIST: As you may know, a psychotherapist can reveal information about someone only with that person's consent. [*I pause to give Gwen time to respond.*]

GWEN: You can't tell me anything?

THERAPIST: No. I am sorry if this is disappointing. I'm going to end this conversation now. Good-bye.

In Example 11.4, I protect Sallie's confidentiality while also treating Gwen with respect and empathy, a winning combination. Interestingly enough, as I have become more comfortable setting and holding limits within a treatment, it has become easier (and more effective) to link a polite attitude with firm limits.

I will inform Sallie of Gwen's call during her next psychotherapy session. Our therapeutic alliance might increase in strength when Sallie learns that I am so vigilant about protecting her privacy.

Even when I have a signed consent to talk to another individual about a patient, I make sure the person on the phone is the person I am authorized to talk to before sharing confidential information. For instance, if Sallie had agreed that I could talk with a school counselor, I would confirm the individual's identity by calling his business number directly before discussing any clinical issues.

THE INSURANCE COMPANY WANTS INFORMATION ABOUT YOUR PATIENT

Sometimes insurance companies request a copy of my patient's outpatient medical record. With rare legal situations as exceptions, I cannot provide any medical information to another party without a release signed by my patient.

If a patient authorizes me to correspond with her insurance company, it is to her benefit if I provide as little personally sensitive information as feasible. Insurance companies aren't innocuous institutions interested solely in a patient's welfare. It is even possible that they could misuse the information they obtain to deny present or future treatment benefits.

Whenever an insurance company asks for a summary of the ongoing treatment, I talk openly with my patient about the information I will include in the report. Some patients are less worried about confidentiality and more concerned that they obtain their full insurance benefits for mental health, no matter what needs to be revealed. Others are not willing to be so open and may end insurance coverage of sessions prematurely in order to protect their privacy. By reviewing with the patient what information needs to be kept private and what can be revealed to the insurance company, the therapeutic alliance will be protected. As always, if I have any doubts, I'll consult supervisors about their recommended strategies in such situations.

YOUR PSYCHIATRIC NOTES ARE SUBPOENAED

A subpoena is a document that requests the presence of a witness or of records before a court. While complete coverage of this topic is beyond the scope of this book, we have outlined a preliminary strategy that we follow if a subpoena requests a patient's psychiatric notes. If faced with this type of situation, we also recommend consulting a supervisor and/or an attorney to review the specifics of your clinical situation.

One example: I receive a subpoena from my patient's ex-husband's lawyer for my patient's psychiatric record. Currently, the couple is battling for custody of their only child. What should I do?

First, I'll call my clinic's or hospital's attorney. If the subpoena is *not* accompanied by the patient's authorization or a court order specifically agreeing to or ordering the release of psychotherapy records, the hospital attorney and I should let the issuer of the subpoena know that I cannot comply because the patient's records are privileged under state law. I will not discuss any details of the records with the ex-husband's attorney.

At my patient's next session, I will inform her of the subpoena and my response to it. I will also call the company providing my professional liability insurance to inform them of the details of the situation.

If the subpoena includes the patient's authorization or a court order, I am required to provide the court with a copy of the patient's official medical psychiatric record. I shall also notify my clinic's attorney and my professional liability insurance company. In this particular situation, it is again an advantage to have two sets of patient notes: the official medical record and my own personal process notes that don't include the patient's name. Personal notes are not official medical record material, and I can provide the court with the patient's medical information without sharing many of her private concerns.

What if the subpoena specifically requests my process notes or broadly requests any and all records related to the patient? If the attorney obtains a court order or the patient's authorization, I may be bound to release my process notes in addition to the medical record. Faced with this type of complication, I would also return to my supervisor and an attorney for more detailed guidance.

To avoid this type of situation, some therapists choose not to keep process notes for therapy cases that have a high likelihood of legal involvement. While this decision is certainly understandable, it's not a simple decision. The absence of notes may make it difficult—at least for some of us—to provide optimal treatment.

Sometimes, my patient may wish to share her psychotherapy records with her attorney. She may hope the information in the notes will help her win her lawsuit, whether it be a custody battle or an insurance dispute. In fact, the release of these records is rarely helpful in a legal sense, and the decision may have many unforeseen negative emotional consequences. Once the psychotherapy file becomes part of the legal record, the opposing side has the opportunity to misuse, misunderstand, or manipulate the information. If I am subpoenaed to testify, I am required under oath to answer all questions accurately, even if that means divulging very private information about the patient. My role as an advocate could be very limited, and the process may affect future treatment if the therapeutic alliance is threatened. If a patient requests a psychological perspective as part of her legal argument, it is legally and therapeutically more secure to obtain an independent consultation with a clinician she will not see for ongoing treatment.

CONFIDENTIALITY MAY BE BROKEN WHEN THE PATIENT IS A DANGER TO HERSELF OR TO OTHERS

There are a few situations in which it is in the best interest of the patient or the greater community for the therapist to disclose privileged information. In an emergency situation, such as when a patient is suicidal, homicidal, or unable to care for herself, a clinician has the right—in fact, the duty—to obtain help. Usually this includes divulging essential information about the patient's condition.

As a beginner, it can be easy to overreact and to bring in an emergency team prematurely when a patient expresses thoughts of suicide or homicide. I make this mistake in Example 11.5 when Candice Jones unexpectedly expresses suicidal and homicidal feelings during a session.

EXAMPLE 11.5

The patient recalls a history of physical abuse, expresses suicidal and homicidal feelings, and the therapist panics

CANDICE: I've never talked to you about this before, but I think I understand now why I am having so much trouble sleeping this month. It's the anniversary month.

THERAPIST: Anniversary of what?

CANDICE: Anniversary of the day I left home to escape my father and live with my aunt in Boston. I was just 16. It should be a happy occasion. I don't know why I always feel so upset around this time of year.

THERAPIST: This sounds like a very distressing memory. What were you escaping from when you went to live with your aunt?

CANDICE: I haven't told you the details about this, but my father used to hit me all the time growing up. I had lots of company. My mother and my sister had to deal with it too.

We didn't tell anyone about it. We all kept the secret together. At a certain point, when I couldn't bear it any longer, I left. (*becoming increasingly agitated as she talks about this topic*)

THERAPIST: [*I am worried about Candice's ability to tolerate these feelings, so I check how Candice is experiencing the discussion.*] What does it feel like to talk about this?

CANDICE: It is infuriating! That man deserves to die for what he did to my family. When I think about it, I just want to kill my father for what he has done. Then, I might as well kill myself also. It would be easier than having to deal with these memories.

THERAPIST: I'm glad you could tell me about this incredibly traumatic time, and I want to learn more about it. I am worried to hear that these memories are so unbearable that you feel like killing your father and yourself. [*I hear increased anxiety in my voice.*]

CANDICE: Well, that's the way it is. That son of a bitch should get what he deserves.

THERAPIST: I am sorry, but if you are at risk of hurting yourself or anyone else I must take you to the emergency room to be evaluated. [*I call hospital security to escort Candice to the emergency room.*]

When Candice becomes overwhelmed with affect, I panic and move into crisis mode before clarifying whether she actually has any true intent or plan to hurt her father or herself. While it is always better to be cautious, my reaction is based on fear rather than on a thorough assessment.

A deeper evaluation would have obtained additional information before leaning toward an emergency room consultation. Figure 11.2 outlines the pertinent questions I need to answer in order to decide whether Candice is safe to leave the office and go home. If Candice doesn't have a history of acting on her destructive feelings (a history of violence is a strong predictor of future violence) and can assert that she doesn't have a current intention or plan to hurt herself or others, it's likely that her threats are solely an expression of her distress.

If I still feel unsure whether Candice or her father is at risk after a more detailed assessment, I would send Candice with an escort for further evaluation in the emergency room. While I will need to share pertinent clinical information with the crisis team, I can still safeguard most of Candice's confidences from our previous sessions. (See Chapter 9 for more information on patients' crises in general.)

Whatever I decide to do, my note will document the details of my suicidal and homicidal assessment and will state the reasoning behind my treatment decision.

Example 11.6 illustrates a strategy I might employ if Candice is suicidal and/or homicidal with intent and a plan.

The therapist can ask, "Have you had a(n) _____?"

	Of others	Of self
Fleeting thought of death		
Passive wish for death		
Active wish for death		
Intent to pursue death		
Plan to pursue death		
Actions to implement the plan for death		

For each of these questions, the therapist can also ask whether the patient has had previous experience with these thoughts, feelings, and actions, and whether alcohol or other psychoactive drugs were involved. These factors increase a patient's present and future risk.

FIGURE 11.2. Suicidal or Homicidal Assessment Chart.

EXAMPLE 11.6

The therapist carefully assesses suicidality or homicidality in a high-risk patient

The scene opens with Candice becoming increasingly agitated as she talks about years of physical abuse by her father.

CANDICE: Dr. Bender, he deserves to be punished for his behavior. He was never legally charged for his crime. I still have chronic knee pain where he kicked me when I was 13. That son of a bitch should die. Someone needs to make him pay for his actions.

THERAPIST: I agree that your father's behavior was reprehensible, but I am also wondering if you have thought about being the one to exact revenge?

CANDICE: I have, in fact. Next week I'll return to Florida to see my mother, and I plan to stop by and see my father. It's time that he suffer the consequences of his actions.

THERAPIST: Make him pay in what kind of way?

CANDICE: Like I said, Dr. Bender, he deserves to die. I'm not worried about jail. Maybe after he's gone, I'll be ready to die too. I haven't decided on the specifics yet.

THERAPIST: Let's think it through together. How would you make him pay?

CANDICE: I don't know. I'm not sure if I'll have the guts to go through with it, but it's definitely what he deserves. I'm not sure what will happen, but I can't promise. . . .

THERAPIST: Promise?

CANDICE: I don't know. I am just thinking about my options.

THERAPIST: Which options have you considered?

CANDICE: I'd rather not say. Let's just pretend I never brought this up.

THERAPIST: It's a lot better for you and for our work together if you talk to me about this openly.

CANDICE: (*increasingly manipulative*) I'm not interested in discussing it anymore.

THERAPIST: We need to talk about this here or, to protect you, we can walk down together to the emergency room downstairs and talk there.

CANDICE: Dr. Bender, I feel you are acting intrusive. This is my private decision, and I would rather not talk about this anymore.

THERAPIST: I hope we can work through this together, but my first priority is for your safety. I'd like to bring in some other clinicians to get additional opinions on this situation. [*I reach for the phone and request security, using a code word to come to my office and to escort Candice to the emergency room.*]

If Candice were cooperative, I'd assess her homicidal impulses toward her father in detail. To protect Candice and her father, I need to know if she is truly planning to hurt her father in the near future by assessing her intent and plan. When Candice becomes increasingly provocative and refuses to answer my questions, I am legally obligated to continue the evaluation until I can adequately assess both her safety and the risk to her father as a potential victim.

I don't need to tell Candice about my legal obligation to protect her father at this point. By managing her distress in a structured setting, I can protect both parties at once. Either Candice and I need to talk until we have formulated an effective and protective treatment plan, or I need to make sure that she is evaluated immediately in an emergency facility

During the emergency room visit, my colleagues and/or I can decide whether Candice is safe to go home or whether she requires hospitalization to protect herself and her father. If Candice has access to a firearm, it should be turned over to the authorities as part of the crisis intervention. I would only contact Candice's father as a last resort, for example, if Candice elopes from treatment. I'd much prefer to contain her with therapeutic means, such as a locked inpatient hospitalization. The program would provide the necessary intensive patient care while protecting the potential victim and preserving the patient's confidentiality.

In Example 11.6, I call the hospital's emergency security number to ask for assistance in moving Candice from the clinic to the psychiatric emergency room. If I were in a private office and I were unable to convince my patient to obtain an emergency assessment, I would consider calling the police to escort my patient to the nearest emergency facility. If my patient flees from the office, I will ask the police to locate her and then to take her to the nearest hospital for an evaluation.

I have the legal responsibility under laws that vary from state to state to protect a potential victim from an impending assault and to report information about a violent crime that might occur in the future. In Massachusetts, and many other states, clinicians are also required to report any potential or ongoing abuse or neglect that puts children, the elderly, or the disabled in harm's way. However, as a therapist, I do not have the responsibility to report details of a crime that has already oc-curred. In fact, this information is protected under the confidentiality agreement of the therapy.

Confidentiality is a complicated issue that pervades all aspects of psychotherapy. As a therapist, I have a fiduciary duty to safeguard a pa-tient's privacy and physical safety. In specific instances, I also have the conflictual duty to disclose information in order to protect the safety of the patient or of other individuals. Each case is unique, and even with some experience with these issues, I have a low threshold to consult a su-pervisor and/or an attorney when new questions emerge.

Key words: communication, confidentiality, consultation, court orders, data storage, disclosure, disguised information, duty to report, electronic data storage, ethics, exceptions, fiduciaries, informed consent, litigation, medical records, patients' access to records, privileged communication, process notes, psychotherapy, psychotherapy records, subpoena, supervision, trust, waivers

Part III

Chemistry

12

Substance Abuse

For a patient struggling with substance abuse, drug-seeking may become the major focus of life, overriding personal relationships and occupational responsibilities. Self-deception and deception of others around issues involving drugs are cardinal aspects of substance abuse.

Early in treatment, a patient with chemical dependence may deny that she has a problem. The interpersonal and situational problems that beset the patient will rarely be resolved effectively while the substance abuse continues.

The psychotherapy of a patient who is actively abusing substances requires some special strategies. Early detection, firm but empathic confrontation, consistent encouragement, and patience in responding to slips and lapses are necessary to help the patient recover.

The comprehensive treatment of patients with substance abuse is a clinical subspecialty. This chapter attempts to provide an introduction for clinicians learning to treat this set of patients.

When I started practicing psychotherapy, I had both the enthusiasm of a true believer and the naiveté of a novice. I believed in the power of psychodynamic psychotherapy to alleviate distress, and I didn't see the need to alter the approach based on the patient's needs. The basic strategy seemed foolproof—every individual would experience sustained emotional growth if he or she had the opportunity to talk about the past and to connect its difficulties with the present.

While my model was well intentioned, it wasn't long before I realized that one treatment modality can't be applied effectively to every patient. When a patient begins to talk about past or current emotional conflicts in psychotherapy, her anxiety level is likely to increase before it subsides. For most patients, this increase in anxiety is relatively short-lived and tolerable, but for patients with less well-honed coping mechanisms, an immediate focus on emotionally stressful material may be destabilizing. This is often the case for the patient who is actively abusing substances.

In response to the flood of feeling that accompanies an intense psychotherapy session, the substance abuser is apt to turn to alcohol or drugs to manage her distress. If the therapy continues to uncover conflicts without calming the patient's increasing dysphoria, the substance abuse and all related difficulties are likely to get worse instead of better. For treatment to be effective for this group of patients, the traditional psychodynamic insight-oriented approach needs to be modified.

To formulate the most effective treatment strategy for a new patient, I try to identify whether she has an active substance abuse problem within the first few visits of the consultation. Doing this takes some clinical finesse, because both nonusers and active users will deny drug consumption when asked about it directly.

In this chapter, we will focus on the treatment of a new hypothetical patient, Mr. Anthony Lee, a 35-year-old business consultant who begins therapy because of increasing feelings of depression over the preceding several months. In Example 12.1, I fail to identify Anthony's active substance abuse problem during my initial assessment.

EXAMPLE 12.1

The therapist does not recognize that her new psychotherapy patient is also an active substance abuser

During the First Three Consultation Meetings

ANTHONY: So, I don't really understand why I feel so down, Doc, but one of my best friends encouraged me to at least try therapy, so here I am. I figured it couldn't hurt.

THERAPIST: I'm glad you took this first step to get some help; it sounds like you have really been suffering. Could you tell me, during this tough time, have you ever tried to drown your sorrows in alcohol or drugs?

ANTHONY: Nah. I just drink with my friends after work. It's part of the business culture. Nothing to really worry about.

THERAPIST: When you drink, how much do you drink?

ANTHONY: Nothing out of the ordinary. Maybe a beer or two at most.

THERAPIST: Okay.

Example 12.2 illustrates how I could clarify my patient's substance abuse more accurately during the consultation.

EXAMPLE 12.2

The therapist identifies her new psychotherapy patient as an active substance abuser

During the First Three Consultation Meetings

THERAPIST: During this tough time, have you tried to drown your sorrows in alcohol or drugs?

ANTHONY: No. I just drink with my friends after work. It's part of the business culture. Nothing to really worry about, Doc.

THERAPIST: When you drink, what is your drink of choice?

ANTHONY: Oh, just beer mainly, especially the local brews made here in Boston. At this point, I'm a bit of a connoisseur, if I say so myself. It's a fun hobby.

THERAPIST: How much beer can you hold down in one sitting? [*I appeal to Anthony's machismo, which may help him to report his actual use rather than to minimize his intake.*]

ANTHONY: Oh, I don't know, maybe two or three beers at a time. If it's a long night, I may have a few more. Nothing to worry about though. It never affects my work performance.

THERAPIST: Can you hold down four to six beers in a few hours?

ANTHONY: Oh, definitely. That's not a problem.

THERAPIST: [*A tolerance for four to six beers at one sitting may be excessive for any individual, but especially for Andrew, who is 5'8" and not obese. This information suggests that his liver has developed an increased capacity to metabolize alcohol. My concern that Anthony may be actively abusing alcohol has increased.*] How often do you go drinking? Every night? [*My guess is purposely high so Anthony won't feel embarrassed in case he is actually drinking that often.*]

ANTHONY: Oh, not that often. Just a few times a week, at the most.

THERAPIST: Including weekends?

ANTHONY: Usually Saturday night—socially—and I might drink a little on Sunday afternoon if there is a football game.

THERAPIST: Have you experimented with any drugs?

ANTHONY: Well, I used to smoke pot in college, but I do that only occasionally at parties these days. I never buy the stuff, but I may take part in the festivities, if you know what I mean. At my work, this is a normal part of the social scene.

THERAPIST: Ever tried any other drugs? Cocaine? Heroin? Pills?

ANTHONY: I've made it a point to stay away from the hard drugs, Doc. Didn't want to get addicted, you know.

Hey, I know you are just doing your job, but I don't think we need to focus on this so intently.

THERAPIST: Right now, I'm just trying to understand what role alcohol and drugs play in your life. All these substances can affect mood and may contribute to the "down" feeling you are describing to me.

I have four questions I ask everyone about alcohol and drug use. I'd like to review them with you now. [*I prepare to review the CAGE questionnaire—a list of four screening questions have been specifically developed to identify surreptitious alcoholics or substance abusers.*]

ANTHONY: Okay.

THERAPIST: [*I ask the first CAGE question.*] Have you ever tried to cut down on your alcohol and/or drug use at any point in your life?

ANTHONY: Well, drugs have never been a big deal for me. I am trying to cut down a little bit on my drinking now, but there's a good reason.

My first year at my consulting firm, I wanted to make a good impression with my boss, and he spends every evening after work in the local pub. I made a special effort to keep him company after hours talking shop, and it paid off. We've got a great relationship, and if I can knock down a few more brewskies than I could last year, well that only makes it easier to keep up with my colleagues on our nights out.

This year though, I am trying to cut down on my pub meetings to about two to three times a week because I've gained a fair amount of weight. Alcohol and chips isn't the greatest diet, I guess. My mother started to worry I was malnourished because my only vegetables were the olives on the bar nachos. Unless you count the ketchup on the burger (*grins*). You know what I mean.

My diet has improved though, and I recently joined a health club near work. So far, this year I'm much healthier than last.

THERAPIST: That sounds like progress in taking better care of yourself. [*I note privately that the answer to Question 1 is yes and move on to Question 2.*] Has anyone ever gotten annoyed at you for your drinking or your drug use at any time in your life?

ANTHONY: Let me think. I don't think so. Most of my friends and business buddies drink as much as or more than I do. Oh, there was one woman I briefly dated last spring who was concerned about my drinking, but I really think she was overreacting. Maybe some of my buddies have a problem, but in contrast, I'm a total lightweight.

THERAPIST: Have you ever been annoyed at someone for bothering you about your drinking?

ANTHONY: I don't think so. Well, maybe I got a little annoyed at Angela, the woman I dated, even though I knew she had my best interests at heart. She did fixate on my drinking; I really think she was overreacting.

THERAPIST: [*I silently note that the answer to Question 2 is yes.*] Have you felt guilty about your drinking or drug use ever in your life?

ANTHONY: Just when Angela kept drawing my attention to it. I liked her a lot, even though I'm complaining about her now. The relationship just petered out after a few months. I think I was too busy to get involved with anyone seriously last year.

THERAPIST: [*I note the answer to Question 3 is yes.*] Do you ever drink or use drugs in the morning to help get you going after a long night of partying?

ANTHONY: Oh, no! I would never do that!

THERAPIST: [*The answer to Question 4 is no.*] This information is important, and may help us understand the depressed feelings you have described to me. The alcohol may be affecting your mood in ways you haven't considered.

In Example 12.2, I use the CAGE questionnaire (C-Cut down, A-Annoyed, G-Guilty, E-Eye-opener) to evaluate Anthony's current alcohol problem. While these four questions were orginally developed to screen for alcohol abuse, I also use them to evaluate any concurrent drug abuse.

The questionnaire purposely avoids questions about quantity or frequency of drug use as most patients will minimize this information. Research has found that if a patient answers "yes" to more than one question on the CAGE questionnaire, there is a greater than 80% chance that he (or she) has a substance abuse problem. With three "yes" answers (like Anthony), nearly all respondents are sufferers from alcohol or drug abuse or dependence. (For more information on the CAGE questionnaire, see Chapter 5.)

Once I've identified substance abuse as a significant problem in a patient's life, I start to strategize. If I don't choose my words carefully when I talk to Anthony about his excessive alcohol use, he may become defensive and withdraw. On the other hand, the treatment will undoubtably suffer if I ignore the fact that he is drinking too much too often.

EXAMPLE 12.3

The therapist confronts her patient about his substance abuse in an authoritative and ultimately nontherapeutic manner and then colludes with the patient to ignore the mounting evidence that the patient has a substance abuse problem

I have just reviewed the CAGE questionnaire (as illustrated in Example 12.2).

THERAPIST: As I think about your answers to my questions about alcohol, I wonder whether you are drinking excessively, and whether this should be our first focus in your treatment.

ANTHONY: Oh, I don't think my drinking is a problem. I don't drink anymore than any of my friends. I don't drink every night. My work reviews have been excellent. Not what you would see with an alcoholic, I would think.

THERAPIST: Have you ever gotten into any trouble with your drinking?

ANTHONY: No, not at all. Doc, I hate to say this, but you may be overreacting because your circle of colleagues has fun in a very different way than mine. I don't see shrinks being the drinking type. My work is different. Socializing is a big part of what I do. I don't think you need to worry. My drinking is not a big deal.

THERAPIST: Why doesn't it feel like a big deal to you?

ANTHONY: Well (*sounding irritated*), because it's not. I don't see how you came to this conclusion in the first place. I'm not at all worried about my drinking.

THERAPIST: (*becoming somewhat authoritative and a little defensive*) Well, I *am* worried about your alcohol use. The questions I asked you have been used for years to screen individuals for alcoholism. The data have shown that if a person answers more than two of the questions affimatively, it is highly likely that a substance abuse problem exists. Now, we can ignore this information, or we can use it to benefit our work together. I'm concerned that if we ignore it, any work that we do would be unlikely to make you feel better. Alcohol is a depressant, and if we don't address your drinking head on, your suffering is likely to continue, or even get worse.

ANTHONY: (*Responds with an offensive approach*) Look Doc, I appreciate your concern, but I came to see you because of the difficulties I have had concentrating at work and this depressed feeling I sometimes get. If anything, alcohol makes me feel better, not worse. I didn't come to you to talk about my social life with my work buddies. My interactions with these guys is one of the few parts of my life that is fun, and it isn't causing any problems.

THERAPIST: [*I feel intimidated and unsure. I don't want to make Anthony more upset than he already is.*] Okay, maybe I'm wrong. Can you tell me about how you view your difficulties?

ANTHONY: Well, it's like this . . .

Anthony becomes more defensive and oppositional when I confront him about his alcohol use in a direct, rather authoritative manner. In an attempt to avoid further conflict and salvage the therapeutic alliance, I switch topics before we reach any mutual understanding about his use of alcohol. Neither strategy helps Anthony consider treatment for his excessive drinking.

Example 12.4 illustrates a more effective way to talk openly but sensitively to a patient in denial about a substance abuse problem.

EXAMPLE 12.4

The therapist sensitively confronts a patient with an active substance abuse problem who is in denial

I've just reviewed the CAGE questionnaire (as illustrated in Example 12.2).

THERAPIST: From what you have said, your drinking sounds risky. It would be in your best interest if we were to start treatment by focusing on this problem.

ANTHONY: Oh, I don't think my drinking is a problem. I don't drink any more than any of my colleagues. I don't drink every night and I don't drink alone. It's more of a social thing.

THERAPIST: I understand that you don't see it as a problem. Maybe you aren't aware of the difficulty yet, but alcohol can cause trouble quickly.

ANTHONY: Nah, I appreciate your concern, Doc, but you don't have to worry. What I'm here for is to understand why I feel depressed most of the time nowadays. If anything, drinking makes me feel better.

THERAPIST: I agree that it is very important to understand why you have been feeling so depressed lately. Many people don't realize that drinking may exacerbate a low mood. Although alcohol can make a person feel better briefly, over time it can act as a chemical depressant, affecting mood in a very negative way. I wouldn't be doing you any favors by ignoring this potential problem.

ANTHONY: I think alcohol has been one of the few joys left in my life, to be honest. What's your point? What would you want me to do differently?

THERAPIST: Well, for starters, would you be willing to have some blood tests? They could give us some indication of whether alcohol has affected your body.

ANTHONY: Sure, but you'll see. I'm sure the tests will be normal. I'm very healthy.

THERAPIST: I hope that's true, but we need to keep a very close eye on this. Have you ever been in any legal trouble related to your alcohol use, or otherwise?

ANTHONY: No, never. See, it's not that bad. I came in for help with my depression. That's my biggest concern at this point.

THERAPIST: It's a very good point. We won't lose sight of the fact you are struggling with depression. [*I make a point to use Anthony's terms to describe his melancholy mood.*]

Because alcohol can act as a depressant, it may help to stop drinking. Alcohol may be making you feel worse in the long run rather than better.

ANTHONY: I don't really understand. A beer after a long day of work just helps me relax. What could be wrong with that?

THERAPIST: As the blood level builds up, alcohol can feel relaxing, but over time, even days later, its chemistry fosters depression.

ANTHONY: Alcohol is the great escape from all my day-to-day pressures. I don't want to give it up.

THERAPIST: This is a worrisome statement. Alcohol seems to be helping you cope during a difficult time, and this can lead to further problems. In therapy, we can try to find ways for you to deal with your worries that don't have such destructive potential.

ANTHONY: You sure are stuck on this point. You really think it's that important?

THERAPIST: I do.

ANTHONY: This just doesn't sound right to me. I'm not an alcoholic; I'm a businessman who drinks. Most of us do.

THERAPIST: What does the the term "alcoholic" mean to you?

ANTHONY: You know the image. The homeless guy asking for a quarter with a bottle inside a brown paper bag. You have to agree. That's not me at all.

THERAPIST: That's certainly not you, but only 3% of alcoholics are on "Skid Row," and the other 97% have other kinds of problems. I'm glad you have been doing so well at work, but from what you have told me, it is likely that the alcohol use may be involved in the depression that is bringing you down.

ANTHONY: Doc, I think you are chasing an issue that really doesn't exist. I don't want my therapy to focus on drinking when it isn't really a problem.

THERAPIST: I understand that you don't see this as a problem, but alcohol can be dangerous the way that you have been using it.

ANTHONY: Boy, you are really serious, I guess. (*Looks a bit upset.*)

THERAPIST: Yes.

ANTHONY: Well, if you really think it's that important, I guess I can get the blood tests and try to stop drinking for a week to see if it helps me feel better.

Example 12.4 illustrates a number of therapeutic tactics a clinician can employ when talking to a patient about a potential substance abuse problem.

First, I concentrate on educating Anthony on the physical and emotional dangers of his current alcohol use, while avoiding a lecturing tone. I don't use phrases such as "I'm very concerned about . . . " or "I'm convinced you have a problem . . . " because they subtly pit my opinions against his beliefs. Instead, my statements review the facts while excluding my opinion within the sentence structure: "Because alcohol can act as a depressant, it may help to stop drinking as alcohol may be making you feel worse in the long run rather than better."

Second, I don't use authoritative phrases such as "You should," "You need to," or "I think that this is definitely the issue here." Instead, my statements refer to the patient's own words: "From what you have said . . . " and "I understand that you don't see this as a problem. . . . " By excluding directive comments, I am more likely to solidify the therapeutic alliance and to make a useful intervention.

For the intervention to work, I need to impart the same message of empathy and concern for an active substance abuser as I might for any other patient. The moment the patient feels that I am judging him unfavorably, his defensiveness will increase, and my ability to be effective will be impaired.

To support this process, it often helps to externalize the substance abuse problem so the patient and I can critically examine it together. Alcohol is personified and discussed as a problem, separate from the person who is drinking it. I use this strategy in Example 12.4 when I comment, "As the blood level builds up, alcohol can feel relaxing, but over time, even days later, its chemistry fosters depression." This statement carries a very different emotional valence than "When *you* drink, *your* alcohol level builds up, and that causes *your* depression to get worse."

By using the cognitive and empathic approaches outlined above, I let Anthony know that it is in his best interest to focus on alcohol use during his treatment. I can order liver function tests (GGTP, SGOT, SGPT, CAMP, alkaline phosphatase, MCV; acronyms are spelled out in the "Key words" section) and a complete blood count to assess whether Anthony has any liver damage associated with his increased alcohol consumption. Anthony could obtain these tests at his primary care physician's (PCP) office or at an outside laboratory. Since non-MD therapists do not have the option of using an outside laboratory for testing, they will need to refer the patient to his PCP for a medical workup.

Once Anthony agrees to discuss his substance abuse openly within the treatment, the therapy should proceed with a slightly different slant from that of a traditional insight-oriented psychotherapy.

EXAMPLE 12.5

Typical therapy session with a substance abuser in the very early stages of recovery

ANTHONY: Doc, it feels like a month since our meeting last week. Damn, it was a difficult week at work!

THERAPIST: (*concerned look*) What happened?

ANTHONY: Well, my boss (Remember the one I told you about who drinks every night? His name is Bruce, by the way.) had some sort of vendetta against me this week. I'm not the only one who has noticed it. While he used to go out of his way to help me out, over the last 7 days he has become obsessed with critiquing my work. I think the greatest joy of his day is pointing out what's wrong with me. It's all I can do to stay calm in the office.

THERAPIST: I can understand that this would be very upsetting. Has he ever done this before?

ANTHONY: Never. In general, I get along with him better than most of my colleagues. I worked so hard to create a place for myself at this firm, this is NOT what I need right now. I hear his ex-wife is in town this week, and maybe that's why he is being such a pisser. Whatever the reason for his attitude, it's making my life impossible.

THERAPIST: How are you feeling?

ANTHONY: I feel like crap. Who wouldn't?

THERAPIST: How are coping with feeling so badly?

ANTHONY: Ummm, well, I went drinking last night with some friends from work and that helped. A little escape can do wonders, you know.

THERAPIST: How much did you drink?

ANTHONY: Not much, just a few beers.

THERAPIST: [*I remember that Anthony is likely to minimize his alcohol intake. Also of note: In the last session he had agreed to abstain from alcohol because it is a mood depressant. Clearly Anthony wasn't able to avoid drinking for even a week.*] How long were you able to keep from drinking since our last session?

ANTHONY: Oh, yeah, I didn't forget our discussion that alcohol could be making my depression worse. I didn't touch the stuff until yesterday. At that point, I needed any pick-me-up I could find. It was a hellish day. Bruce was impossible.

THERAPIST: You wanted to drink because it helped distract you after Bruce was so unreasonable?

ANTHONY: Yes, but so what? A lot of people have a drink or two after a hard day at work.

THERAPIST: How do you think alcohol helped you to feel better?

ANTHONY: Well, I was so angry and the beers helped me feel mellow and back to normal. It was such a relief to take a break from the stress and have some fun.

THERAPIST: The conflict with Bruce is very stressful.

ANTHONY: Yeah, it is.

THERAPIST: I agree that it is very important to have a way to relieve your stress after dealing with Bruce. Alcohol seems to work in the short term, but it will ultimately increase your level of stress by exacerbating your depression.

Maybe we need to think together about other strategies that will help you cope with Bruce without worsening your depression.

ANTHONY: What do you mean?

THERAPIST: Can you think of other ways to release stress other than drinking?

ANTHONY: Well, I feel better after I work out.

THERAPIST: Working out is a great way to feel better, and it improves physical and emotional health. How often do you exercise?

ANTHONY: I try to go to the gym a couple times a week, but work has been too busy lately, so I haven't been able to go for a while.

THERAPIST: If you aren't able to make it to the gym, what other ways can you decrease your stress?

ANTHONY: Other than drinking?

THERAPIST: Yes.

ANTHONY: Umm, well, I do like to watch sports, especially football.

THERAPIST: But you told me you drink beer on Sundays when you watch football.

ANTHONY: But that would be easy to give up. The sport itself is like a drug for me. I love it so much.

THERAPIST: Why football specifically?

ANTHONY: I played in high school and in intramurals in college. I was the quarterback both times.

THERAPIST: Are they good memories?

ATHONY: Yeah. I'm too small to be really good, but I love the game. Plus, when I was playing often, I was in good shape and hung around with some great guys. They are still some of my best friends.

THERAPIST: How would it feel to try these two activities—working out and watching sports—instead of drinking this week when you feel stressed?

ANTHONY: Sure. I'll give it a try.

During the next 2 months, Anthony and I discuss many different adaptive mechanisms to help him deal with stress. During each discussion, he seems interested in trying new alternative coping mechanisms, such as imagery, music, or social activities, that don't involve alcohol.

However, he admits that he continues to drink heavily and frequently. It is time to talk about Alcoholics Anonymous (AA) to augment his current treatment plan.

Midway into Our Next Session

THERAPIST: When alcohol is used to help with emotional pain, it can end up causing more problems than it helps. Often, it can be helpful to talk to others who have coped with similar difficulties and hear what other methods they have discovered that don't involve drinking.

ANTHONY: Where would I do that?

THERAPIST: I have a list of Alcoholics Anonymous meetings that meet in the financial district and attract people in professions that are fast-paced like yours. What would you think about attending one?

ANTHONY: WHOA! This is too much! I had a night out with my friends last night, but I am not an alcoholic, and NO WAY am I going to an AA meeting! Look, I know this is on the top of your agenda, but I think your focus on my alcohol use is more annoying than therapeutic.

THERAPIST: I don't intend to annoy you, but I understand how our differences of opinion can have that effect. It has been difficult for you to give up drinking these past months. Doesn't that concern you?

ANTHONY: Look, if that's what you are worried about, then I'll just stop drinking, cold turkey. I'd rather stop drinking altogether than to have to keep returning to alcohol as a central topic.

THERAPIST: Okay, let's see if you are able to stop cold turkey one more time. But if you are unable to stop drinking altogether, then I think it will be time to start recognizing the hold that alcohol has on you.

ANTHONY: Okay, if I don't stop. . . . But when I do, you'll see that you have worried unnecessarily. Don't get me wrong. I appreciate your concern. I just think it is misplaced. And I don't see any AA meetings in my future . . . ever.

THERAPIST: That would be your decision, of course, but I hope that the meetings won't be seen as a punishment but rather as the next indicated step in treatment. I wouldn't be providing good care for you if I just ignored the alcohol problem.

ANTHONY: Yeah, well it's a non-issue. No more alcohol use for me, period. I'm always up to a challenge. I don't think it will be that difficult.

THERAPIST: I would have no trouble being proven wrong, but you need to let me know if you do drink again.

ANTHONY: Sure, I think that is fair.

THERAPIST: Let's take it step by step together and see what happens. I think we should continue to try to find other methods that help you to feel better and to improve your depression.

The discussion in Example 12.5 is much more structured than some of the other therapeutic interchanges modeled in this book. First, when Anthony starts talking about his current difficulties with Bruce, I don't delve deeply into his feelings about this relationship. I purposely avoid questions that might evoke an intense reaction, such as "Can you tell me more details of what you feel when Bruce criticizes you?" or "Does he remind you of anyone else in your life from the past?"

These explorations can come later, after Anthony has some healthful coping mechanisms in place. To conquer Anthony's ongoing substance abuse, we spend our time recognizing the events that trigger alcohol use, strategizing how to reduce or avoid these events when possible, and introducing alternative coping methods.

Bruce's treatment of Anthony is a good example of the social pressures that oppose sobriety. Often, people drink when they feel lonely or misunderstood, and a social structure of other heavy drinkers supports the habit. Becoming sober may become more difficult if Anthony loses his special social connection with his boss when his alcohol consumption decreases.

When Anthony's drinking continues unabated, I introduce AA as a possible adjunctive treatment. AA supports sobriety because it provides ongoing contact with sober people in recovery who help the patient battle loneliness without alcohol or drugs. It adds what a patient with excessive drug use may be unconsciously seeking: the soothing effect of social support combined with techniques to fight addiction.

When Anthony balks at this recommendation, I agree to his challenge to pursue abstinence one more time. It is a no-lose proposition: Either Anthony's drinking subsides or he will have new insight into the severity of his substance abuse when he is unable to abstain. The treatment alliance is reinforced, and the patient's needs are protected.

Psychotherapy with active substance abusers is slow work. If Anthony continues to avoid additional substance abuse treatment, such as AA, medications to reduce his desire for alcohol, or alcohol abuse clinics, I will continue to analyze his resistance in a supportive empathic manner. If his drinking escalates and he begins to endanger himself or others, I might start to recommend a more intensive intervention, such as day treatment or an inpatient stay, as the next therapeutic step.

ANTISOCIAL BEHAVIOR IN ACTIVE SUBSTANCE ABUSERS

Active substance abusers also require a special therapeutic touch because they are likely to exhibit comorbid antisocial behaviors. Such behaviors might not remit until the patients have been abstinent for a prolonged period of time. It makes some psychological sense: If a person is ashamed of her substance use but is also psychologically and/or physically addicted to a drug, deceptive behavior patterns are likely to follow. It's not unusual for active users to lie, to minimize their drug use, and to pursue illegal behaviors (stealing) to obtain more of the drug. In fact, whenever I have any suspicion that substance abuse may be an issue, I make a point of asking the patient if she has had any troubles with the law.

Often, the deception that affects the active user's relationships with her family and friends eventually infects the user's relationship with her therapist. When a patient relapses multiple times, she is unlikely to confess to each incident and may lie or minimize her substance use. As the therapist, I'm most effective in this situation if I maintain a sensitive but extremely firm therapeutic stance. Early in treatment, I may rely on the patient's report to track substance abuse. At the first signs of dishonesty, I'll either ask for corroborated information from a significant person in the patient's life or introduce other methods, such as urine screens, to monitor drug intake objectively.

As a naive beginner, I had a humbling experience treating an active substance abuser with a substantial antisocial streak. I saw the patient, whom I'll call Roy, in weekly substance abuse/psychopharmacology sessions for about 6 months. He was an aspiring artist in his early 20s who had been an active heroin abuser for about a year when circumstances led him to seek treatment at the clinic. He adamantly denied any prior substance abuse during his adolescence. Despite my repeated attempts to focus the treatment on his heroin use, he identified depression and anxiety as his primary problems. We compromised by talking about both.

At first, the treatment seemed like a success in the making, and I was pleased with Roy's progress. Within the first few months of treatment, he moved away from the neighborhood in which his heroin-abusing friends congregated. He agreed to attend two Narcotics Anonymous (NA) meetings a week. I didn't ask for written proof of attendance, since he related the details of each meeting during our sessions.

Then, after approximately 30 days of sobriety, he relapsed. I recommended that he start additional counseling from a substance abuse specialist to supplement our weekly meetings. He was reluctant to pursue this, but after 2 more weeks of active using, I insisted that he add this to his treatment program. I also asked that he allow open communication among his various treaters in order to facilitate comprehensive care. He agreed, although without a lot of enthusiasm. He reported the next week that he had started seeing a clinician, "Morgan Murphy," at the MGH's substance abuse specialty clinic.

According to Roy, he was sober at this point, but he continued to complain of newly emerging difficulties in his relationships with his family and friends. He complained that no one understood him. Everyone was judging him. He didn't feel he could trust anyone in his life. I wondered whether he had relapsed, and I called the substance abuse specialty clinic in order to discuss my concerns with Ms. Murphy.

I quickly discovered that Ms. Murphy did not exist, and that Roy had only attended one assessment visit at that clinic. They hadn't seen him for weeks. When I mentioned this to Roy, he also confessed that he had stopped going to his twice weekly NA meetings months ago. He was a little embarrassed at being exposed, but he kept repeating that he hadn't been interested in seeing the substance abuse counselor in the first place. A toxicology screen was positive for heroin metabolites.

I was naive to trust that Roy would tell me the truth about his addiction. Still, I felt foolish and furious after I learned that Ms. Murphy existed only in fantasy. I had a taste of the deception that Roy's family and friends coped with on a daily basis.

As Roy's clinician, I needed to understand my first reaction, but then to respond in a way that was therapeutic, rather than impulsive or angry. I turned to Dr. Messner for supervision, and we worked together to set up a treatment protocol that would acknowledge Roy's vulnerability but protect the therapy from a similar deception in the future. It's a fine line we walk as therapists: trying to understand without condoning self-destructive behavior.

My confrontation with Roy went something like this:

EXAMPLE 12.6

Confronting an active substance abuser who has been lying about his treatment compliance

Moments after I Tell Roy That I Discovered "Morgan Murphy" Doesn't Exist

THERAPIST: If you lie about something to your doctor, it must be very precious to you.

ROY: Look, Dr. Bender, I am really sorry. I kept intending to go to that clinic, but I like you as my therapist. I didn't want to see anyone else.

THERAPIST: Psychotherapy depends upon truth. Unless we are honest with one another, we aren't really conducting psychotherapy, and your distress is unlikely to improve with treatment.

ROY: I'm sorry I lied to you. I'll try to tell you the truth from now on.

THERAPIST: I am glad you feel comfortable working with me, but because heroin addiction is so powerful, your treatment should include additional supports, such as NA meetings and work with the substance abuse clinic. I will continue to work with you as we have been doing if these extra supports are in place.

ROY: Well, I'm not really using that much that often anymore. The last time was about 2 weeks ago. I think I can taper off. I've got the message now, and I promise that I'll tell the truth to you from now on.

THERAPIST: [*I remember that Roy is probably lying.*] If an emotionally difficult situation presents itself, your first impulse is to use drugs and then to deny it.

ROY: Only now and then. Not always.

THERAPIST: I'm glad you aren't using all the time, but heroin is so addicting I think you need to follow a new treatment plan in order for our work to have a fighting chance.

ROY: What do you mean?

THERAPIST: In order for us to work together weekly in psychotherapy, you need to have weekly urine toxicology screens, confirmation of substance abuse meetings and weekly individual meetings with a substance abuse counselor. From now on, I plan to be in touch with your counselor on a regular basis.

ROY: Are you kidding? I don't want to do all that stuff.

THERAPIST: Apparently we disagree, so we might need some time to resolve our differences. I'd like to discuss it with you for a month or two. After 4–8 weeks, you'll need to comply with this treatment plan if we are to continue working together in psychotherapy.

ROY: Well, what if I refuse to do it?

THERAPIST: Of course, that is your choice, but then our weekly work together would end for the time being. I'll continue to see you every 4–6 weeks to monitor your medications.

If you'd like to transfer your care elsewhere, I can provide you with the names of other clinics. For emergencies, you will need to go to your local psychiatric emergency room or to the one at this hospital.

ROY: Why are you doing this to me?

THERAPIST: If I am to work with you in psychotherapy, I need to know that your addiction is also being treated aggressively. I don't want to stand around ignoring the problem while your increasing use could lead to serious injury or death. I can't make you stop using, but I also don't want to support your addiction.

ROY: But you are my doctor. You can't just leave me like this.

THERAPIST: If you won't comply with the treatment contract, I am unwilling to act as your psychotherapist, but I will continue as your psychopharmacologist.

ROY: Ha! You sound like you are trying to get rid of me.

THERAPIST: Not at all. I'm offering 4–8 sessions for us to discuss the new treatment plan. As we talk about the addiction, you may recognize that the new approach has the best chance of helping you recover. If you still refuse to do it, we'll only meet intermittently regarding your medications. Maybe, over time, you'll make some progress recognizing the substance abuse problem. [*I externalize "the problem" as outside of Roy, which makes it more tolerable and less shaming.*]

With 20:20 hindsight, I realize that I should have insisted early on that Roy provide me with objective evidence of attendance in the adjunctive treatment programs. I might have also considered frequent urine toxicology screens from the treatment's beginning. Another important addition to the treatment would be patient-authorized contact between the clinician and someone in the patient's life—a spouse partner, relative, or friend—to monitor clinical progress. With a less impaired patient, it might make sense to start with a more trusting policy. With a patient struggling with a severe addiction, a structured approach is necessary from the start.

Roy and I continued to work together for 2 months after the confrontation illustrated in Example 12.6. He continued to deny the severity of his substance abuse and insisted that his relapse was just temporary. After repeated reminders, I followed through with my plan and ended therapy for the time being. Therapists, just like family and friends, can enable active substance abuse by ignoring its severity.

Unfortunately, after the therapy ended, Roy dropped out of treatment altogether. Roy decided not to meet with me on an intermittent check-in basis. Following Dr. Messner's suggestion, I sent him a letter by certified mail with a return receipt, letting him know he was welcome back for medication treatment. He didn't respond. Evidently, he still wasn't ready for any substance abuse treatment.

Clearly, treating patients struggling with active substance abuse requires special clinical skill. Because their treatment is specialized and complicated, we recommend that your supervisor for these patients be an expert or at least be richly experienced in the treatment of active addiction. He or she will teach you when and how to guide patients toward the different treatment options available (AA and NA meetings, detoxification centers, inpatient hospitalization, psychopharmacological options, and partial day programs).

The clinical recovery of an active substance abuser takes much patience and determination on the part of the therapist as well as powerful motivation on the part of the patient. With an empathic attitude and a sensitive but insistent identification of the emotional triggers that lead to active use, the therapist can help the patient learn when she is at risk. Over time, more healthful coping mechanisms can be put into place. After the patient has at least 6–12 months of continuous sobriety, the therapist can cautiously try a more open-ended psychotherapeutic approach. With some sober supports in place, the patient may be able to tolerate a more insight-oriented psychotherapy and the increased affect that might emerge in its wake.

> **Key words:** Alcoholics Anonymous (AA), alkaline phosphatase, cyclic adenosine monophosphate (CAMP), CAGE questionnaire, detoxification, diagnosis, drug counseling, gamma glutamyl transpeptidase (GGTP), mean corpuscular volume (MCV), Narcotics Anonymous (NA), Rational Recovery, serum glutamic oxaloacetic transaminase (SGOT), serum glutamic pyruvic transaminase (SGPT), twelve-step programs

13

Integrating Psychopharmacology with Psychotherapy

Either an overeager drive in favor of medications or a bias against their use may interfere with optimal psychiatric treatment. If psychotropic medications are indicated, the clinician needs to talk to her patient about the risks and benefits of the treatment and to respond to any concerns the patient may have. Appropriately prescribed medication may enable the depressed, panicky, manic, or psychotic patient to engage more meaningfully in the work of psychotherapy. Depending on the specifics of the clinical situation, it may be preferable to have separate treaters provide the medication and the psychotherapy.

As an undergraduate majoring in psychology, I debated the impact of nature versus nurture on human behavior. As a psychiatrist, I view the two as inextricably intertwined. Experiences affect biology, and biological changes may affect experiences. For example, the complex alterations in brain chemistry seen in clinical depression may affect a person's ability to relate to others. The converse is also true. Emotional events from birth onward have an impact on brain development. It makes sense that comprehensive psychiatric treatment may include both biological (medication, electroconvulsive therapy [ECT], or others) and psychological (the psychotherapies) interventions.

Psychotherapeutic and pharmacological treatments ought to enrich one another. The detailed understanding of the patient derived from psychotherapy can inform the choice of medication. Meanwhile, when psychiatric symptoms endanger life, the appropriate medications can accelerate recovery and enhance the psychotherapeutic process.

Some psychodynamic therapists worry that the introduction of medications will alter the transference in a countertherapeutic manner.

Patients might leave psychotherapy prematurely once they feel some symptomatic relief. Traditionalists believe that the patient may have more difficulty transferring her feelings from other important relationships onto the therapist when the clinician assumes a directive, rather than neutral, stance around psychopharmacological issues.

As a graduate psychoanalyst and a prescriber of medicine for more than 30 years, Dr. Messner has found (as I have with my increasing experience) that an effective and empathic psychopharmacological intervention will nearly always help a therapy to evolve. As the patient feels understood and experiences some relief through the medications, the therapeutic alliance will be enhanced. With increased emotional stability, the patient may be less distracted by her symptoms and more able to talk meaningfully about all issues. The transference will become more accessible to the therapy rather than less. (For more about transference, see Chapter 16.)

Table 13.1 lists a range of psychiatric symptoms that are associated with some of the Axis I disorders in DSM-IV. If a patient's ability to function is substantially and repeatedly impaired by even a few of the symptoms listed, we recommend a psychopharmacological evaluation in conjunction with psychotherapy.

When I am prescribing medications for a patient who sees another clinician for psychotherapy, I'll ask both the patient and the referring therapist for specific details about the recent increase in troublesome symptoms as part of my assessment. The information may highlight troublesome target symptoms and help me to choose the appropriate psychotropic medication.

HOW PSYCHOTHERAPY MAY BE AFFECTED BY THE INTRODUCTION OF MEDICATIONS

Elaine Barber, a new fictitious patient, will illustrate some of the clinical dilemmas that may emerge when a psychotherapy patient is started on medications. Elaine is a 32-year-old single high school English teacher who only suffers from a few mild symptoms of depression when we first start working together. We begin insight-oriented psychodynamic psychotherapy once a week. As treatment progresses over a few months, Ms. Barber experiences a progressive decline in functioning with an increase in dysphoric symptoms. As her psychotherapy continues, it becomes necessary to reassess whether she may need psychotropic medications.

Example 13.1 exaggerates a mistake I made again and again before I became comfortable acting as therapist and psychopharmacologist

TABLE 13.1. Target Symptoms That May Be Improved with Psychopharmacological Treatment

Mood disorders

Symptoms of major depression

Disturbances of sleep, interest, energy, appetite, concentration, with concurrent depressed mood and/or irritability, and possibly suicidality

Symptoms of a variant of bipolar disorder

Distractibility, impulsivity, grandiosity, flight of ideas, increased activity, decreased sleep, and talkativeness

Thought disorders

Delusions, hallucinations, disorganized speech, disorganized behavior, or severe withdrawal

Anxiety disorders

Panic attacks with or without agoraphobia, persistent inhibiting fear in social situations, recurrent distressing obsessions or compulsions that affect the patient's ability to function

Posttraumatic stress symptoms including flashbacks, nightmares, avoidance of stimuli associated with the trauma, general numbing of affect, hypervigilance, or irritability

Eating disorders

Bulimia: binge eating followed by purging (self-induced vomiting or abuse of laxatives)

Substance use disorders

Craving for or excessive consumption of alcohol or drugs

---

simultaneously. Early on, I'd worry that my therapy patient would feel annoyed if I spent precious minutes running through psychopharmacological questions, even if it were clear that she would benefit from a psychotropic medication. To return to a discussion of psychosocial issues, I'd rush through my inquiry as quickly as possible.

EXAMPLE 13.1

The therapist does not complete a thorough
psychopharmacological evaluation for a psychotherapy patient

ELAINE: Dr. Bender, while I've enjoyed talking to you, I must admit that I don't think the therapy is helping me. I've been seeing you once a week for a few months now, and over the last 3 weeks or so, I've started to feel worse instead of better. I am only sleeping a few hours a night now, and I am exhausted at work. I'm barely functioning during the day.

THERAPIST: You have really been suffering. Is your appetite also affected?

ELAINE: Not really. I just don't feel hungry.

THERAPIST: I think we should discuss starting some medication that could help you with these symptoms. It sounds like your symptoms have progressed over the last few months so they are now consistent with a diagnosis of major depression. Here is a prescription for paroxetine. Start taking one pill a day and you will begin to feel better in a month or so. Now, let's think together if there are any stressors that could also be making things more difficult now.

ELAINE: Well, in general, I feel lonely all the time. But wait, I'm not sure I want to take a pill.

THERAPIST: Okay. You don't need to start the medicine right away. We can wait and see if you feel better as we learn more about the loneliness. Can you tell me more?

In Example 13.1, I rush through the psychopharmacology evaluation in order to talk to Elaine in more detail about her loneliness. The review of psychiatric symptoms isn't complete, and the risk of suicide is overlooked. I also don't inform Elaine of any of the risks, specific benefits, and possible side effects that may occur with paroxetine treatment. In fact, this evaluation borders on medical negligence.

Example 13.2 illustrates a more complete approach that balances a psychopharmacological and a psychotherapeutic perspective.

EXAMPLE 13.2

How to talk to a psychotherapy patient about starting medications

Elaine begins as in Example 13.1.

ELAINE: Dr Bender. . . . I'm barely functioning during the day.

THERAPIST: It sounds like things have gotten more difficult instead of easier. When did you notice the change?

ELAINE: Well, everything seems to have become just unbearable over the last few weeks. I'm not sleeping at all any more. I've never felt this horrible before.

THERAPIST: Clearly, we need to pay special attention to these problems right away. Any idea of what might be making things worse?

ELAINE: No, it is a mystery to me. I feel upset most of the time, and I don't even have a good idea why.

THERAPIST: I can imagine that would be very upsetting. Let's take a little time and see if we can try to understand this together.

Because you have been feeling so low, it is possible you may have a major depression. May I ask you a few questions to get more information about your current symptoms?

ELAINE: That would be fine.

THERAPIST: You mentioned that your sleep has been troublesome. In general, how many hours of sleep have you been getting?

ELAINE: Oh, I don't know, not enough. Maybe 2 or 3 hours on average.

THERAPIST: It would be very difficult to function on such little sleep. Have you missed any days of work?

ELAINE: Last week, I stayed home on Wednesday because I just couldn't manage to haul myself out of bed. That's unusual though. In general, I've been going to work.

THERAPIST: [*briefly screening for history of mania in case I hadn't done so during the consultation*] Have you ever experienced any time in your life where you didn't need much sleep but felt unusually energetic and very productive at work?

ELAINE: No, I've never had anything like that. I've always been very sensitive to sleep deprivation. That's why I am so exhausted these days.

THERAPIST: During the last few weeks, has your appetite been affected?

ELAINE: I hadn't really noticed this, but now that you mention it, I haven't been very hungry lately. Food just doesn't look interesting anymore.

THERAPIST: Have you lost any weight?

ELAINE: I'm not sure, but my clothes do feel a little more loose. I didn't notice until you asked.

THERAPIST: Have you been able to concentrate at work even though you have been feeling so badly?

ELAINE: Of course not! (*with an irritable tone*) It's impossible to function adequately on so little food and little sleep. I don't know if my students have noticed that I am acting strangely, but I'm sure they will soon. I used to feel energized when I left work, and now I'm exhausted before lunch time. I can't cope with this much longer! I don't know what is happening to me.

THERAPIST: The symptoms you are suffering from are classic indicators of an illness called major depression. As you are experiencing it, major depression is very serious because its symptoms are so debilitating. Sometimes when someone is having such a tough time, thoughts of suicide come up as well. Has this happened to you?

ELAINE: Sure, sometimes I think about it, but I don't think I would act on it. Not at this point anyway.

THERAPIST: What do you think about?

ELAINE: When I am feeling very low, I imagine jumping in front of a car or out of a window—something like that. But it's just a passing thought. I don't think I could ever act on it, at least not yet. I still have hope that I'll feel better someday.

THERAPIST: I think there are a number of treatment options that may help you, but first let's talk a bit more about your safety. If you ever have a change of heart and want to hurt yourself, would you call me right away or find your way to the nearest emergency room if we weren't able to connect immediately?

ELAINE: I think so.

THERAPIST: Do you promise?

ELAINE: Yes, yes, I don't want to die. But I don't want to feel like this anymore either. Is there anything you can do to help me?

THERAPIST: Yes: prescribe medications. Major depression can be viewed as a chemical imbalance in the central nervous system. Medications can return the imbalance back to normal and alleviate a number of distressing symptoms usually within about 2 to 4 weeks.

ELAINE: Two weeks is a long time.

THERAPIST: It is a long time, especially since you have been feeling poorly for a number of weeks already. Some of the symptoms, such as your difficulty sleeping, might improve even sooner.

ELAINE: But I heard that some of these antidepressants either act like a happy pill and change your personality or work the other way and make you suicidal. I don't want a pill that affects how my mind works.

THERAPIST: Can you tell me more about your concerns?

ELAINE: Well, is it true? I don't want to turn into a Pollyannna and feel happy about things that are upsetting, and I don't want to become more suicidal than I already am. I'm not comfortable with the idea that a drug might change the way I see the world.

THERAPIST: I am glad you bring up these questions. It is a common worry that an antidepressant will change a person's personality or make her a "Pollyanna." Luckily, this isn't the case. The medications help diminish the symptoms I reviewed with you: trouble sleeping, eating, concentrating, and feeling motivated. The very low feeling and intermittent suicidal thoughts should also improve with treatment, but the medicine won't shield you from the ups and downs of everyday life.

ELAINE: But what about this news story I heard a long time ago that these medications made some people suicidal?

THERAPIST: When the first of the new antidepressants came on the market, there was concern that it might be associated with an increased suicide rate. Since then, this claim has not been supported. In fact, according to extensive research on the subject, none of these new antidepressants have been associated with an increase in suicides. On the contrary, antidepressant treatment reduces the risk of suicide.

ELAINE: I feel so low I think I am ready to try anything. You really think it is a good idea?

THERAPIST: I do. You are suffering from symptoms that can usually be treated effectively and safely. But, now, before I know which medicine to recommend, I need to ask you a few more questions about your medical history.

ELAINE: Fine, but this whole process still makes me nervous.

THERAPIST: What makes you nervous about it?

ELAINE: I'm concerned what this might mean about my brain. Am I so weak that I can't tolerate the basic stressors of life?

THERAPIST: I think the best way to think about major depression is to compare it to other diseases that sometimes require medication to improve. If you had diabetes, high blood pressure, or asthma, you probably would not consider your illness a sign of weakness. The type of depression you have is also an illness. It's different from the blue mood people get when they had a bad day. In a way, you already know this because you can feel that this state is so different from anything else you've ever experienced.

ELAINE: I still feel very odd about taking a medicine that will change the way my mind functions.

THERAPIST: Research shows that when a person is depressed, the chemical balance in her brain is abnormally altered. The medications actually return these chemical changes and your brain function to their normal predepression state.

ELAINE: It's possible I have a weak character. Otherwise, I would be able to make myself feel better.

THERAPIST: It is the depression itself that makes a person feel weak. The illness isn't a reflection on your character.

ELAINE: It's true that I haven't been feeling myself lately.

THERAPIST: It's clear that it has been very hard on you to suffer like this.

ELAINE: (*Nods tearfully.*)

THERAPIST: Well, I think it is crucial that we continue to talk about this openly and approach the problem as a team.

ELAINE: Okay.

My interview in Example 13.2 balances psychopharmacological and psychotherapeutic approaches. Before I recommend a medication trial, I complete a structured interview to clarify Elaine's diagnosis and to evaluate her safety. While my approach is more focused and cognitive than during a typical therapy hour, I make sure to leave ample time to discuss Elaine's misgivings about psychotropic medications.

As Elaine lists a number of neurovegetative symptoms that are impairing her daily ability to function (such as decreases in sleep, energy, concentration, appetite, and ability to experience pleasure, accompanied by an intensification of depressed mood, hopelessness, and suicidality), it becomes clear that she is suffering from major depression. I confirm once again that she does not have any history of mania. (Antidepressants given to patients with bipolar disease might instigate a manic reaction.) Antidepressants should provide her with substantial relief.

One might argue: "Maybe Elaine hasn't had enough time to benefit from therapy. If you just gave her more time to talk about the problems in her life, her condition might improve without medications." Elaine's symptoms may also improve with long-term therapy, but we believe that she needs a more aggressive approach as her functioning declines and her risk of suicide increases. A medication trial is clinically indicated.

Before writing out a prescription, I would inform Elaine of the adverse effects and benefits of the recommended medication. I would review the common side effects with her, as well as what to do if any of the side effects occurred between sessions.

Note that the use of paroxetine as the medication mentioned in these examples does not represent a general clinical recommendation. Paroxetine is a member of a class of antidepressants called selective serotonin reuptake inhibitors (SSRIs). Other excellent, efficacious, and safe members of this class include citalopram, fluoxetine, sertraline, and others.

INFLUENCES OF PSYCHOTROPIC MEDICATION ON THE THERAPEUTIC RELATIONSHIP

While psychopharmacological treatment will not hinder the psychotherapeutic process, therapy does change with the introduction of a prescription. If I am acting as both therapist and psychopharmacologist, I need to balance the open forum of psychotherapy with the more structured medical evaluation. Once the patient starts taking the medication, I need to inquire about efficacy and side effects on a regular basis. Some clinicians formalize this arrangement as part of the treatment and set aside some time each month or at each prescription refill to follow-up on psychopharmacological issues.

With experience, it has become second nature to balance the two clinical roles. As a novice therapist though, I found it difficult to juggle the two approaches. Once I had prescribed medication for a patient, I was at risk of attributing any future symptoms to dosages or side effects. Example 13.3 illustrates how it's possible for the psychopharmacological "hat" to get stuck on the prescribing therapist's head.

EXAMPLE 13.3

The therapist becomes too medically oriented after the patient starts taking a medication

Elaine has been taking paroxetine for treatment of a major depression for approximately a month.

ELAINE: I've been feelng better since taking the paroxetine—until yesterday that is.

THERAPIST: (*concerned look*) What happened?

ELAINE: Well, I was just thinking a couple days ago how I've been feeling so much better the last few weeks. But, then yesterday, I was unable to function again. I'm concerned that maybe the medication isn't working after all.

THERAPIST: This sounds upsetting. Can you tell me more about what felt so bad?

ELAINE: Last night I tossed and turned for hours. I think I only slept 3 hours last night.

THERAPIST: How is your appetite?

ELAINE: Well, it was a little better, but then last night I felt so nauseated that I skipped dinner completely.

THERAPIST: Let me ask you a few more questions. We may need to increase the medicine.

ELAINE: Oh, I was wondering about that also.

It is notable that Elaine had been feeling much better until the night before our appointment. Usually, antidepressants don't change efficacy from day to day. In this example, I don't ask many detailed questions about Elaine's change in mood, but prematurely jump to a review of her current neurovegetative symptoms. This is an oversight. Maybe something upsetting occurred yesterday that can explain Elaine's renewed difficulties.

It isn't unusual for a patient who has just started on medication to attribute any new emotional distress to "the depression," ignoring any psychosocial issues that may be involved. It's easy to collude with this approach, as I did in Example 13.3. Manipulation of medication doses may be simpler for both parties than the empathic detective work necessary to understand a psychological reaction.

Example 13.4 illustrates how Elaine's concerns could be addressed with a combined biological and psychological perspective.

EXAMPLE 13.4

When the psychotherapist incorporates both biological and psychological perspectives

Elaine has been taking paroxetine for treatment of a major depression for about a month.

ELAINE: Well, I was feeling better for a time, but now I feel worse again. The medication is no longer working.

THERAPIST: It's always difficult when things take a turn for the worse. Can you tell me what happened?

ELAINE: Well, yesterday, the day seemed to be progressing fine but then all of sudden, I just felt like crying.

THERAPIST: Hmm, any understanding of what could have made you feel so sad?

ELAINE: No . . . not really. I must need a higher dose of medication.

THERAPIST: I think it will be important to review your progress on the paroxetine, but let's try to understand when the terrible feeling started.

ELAINE: I think I was fine until lunch, and then all my energy seeped out of me, and I left work early to go to bed. I felt exhausted. And then, last night, even though I was extremely tired, I still couldn't go to sleep. Dr. Bender (*voice becomes more panicked*), I cannot return to the way I was feeling before. Couldn't you just increase the medication?

THERAPIST: We can consider that option together, but first can you tell me what went on at lunch yesterday? Did anything upsetting happen?

ELAINE: Well, the talk I had with Agnes really upset me. I don't know if I've told you about Agnes before. She has worked as a teacher's aide in my classroom as part of an internship before she receives her teaching degree. She has been just wonderful to work with.

She had heard some gossip from some of the other teachers that she shared with me yesterday. We have a new principal this year. She has been friendly, but no one knows what type of agenda she might have.

According to Agnes, she wants to restructure the entire English department. She feels the students need to have an understanding of all the classic texts, and wants to emphasize this in a revamped curriculum. I don't like this idea, especially because my favorite class to teach is Modern American Literature.

Then, Agnes told me that Irene (*the principal*) may want to cancel my creative writing class as well. This is a class that I have taught for over 5 years. The kids love it. I love it. I don't know why she would do that, but it would be a great loss for me. At this point, this information is just gossip, so I don't feel comfortable asking Irene if it is actually going to take place.

THERAPIST: How did it affect you to hear this news?

ELAINE: I felt terrible. Up until now, I have felt so free and supported at my school. If this is true, my whole experience at the school may change in a fundamental way.

The writing class was my creation, and it is very popular among the students. The class is my favorite hour of the day. I become very close to the students. Teaching wouldn't be as fulfilling if I'm not allowed to offer this elective. If Agnes is right, this is very depressing news.

THERAPIST: (*Nods, with encouraging eye contact with Elaine.*)

ELAINE: And this time of the year is especially heinous for me.

THERAPIST: How so?

ELAINE: Well, it's November 2nd today. In just a few weeks it will be Thanksgiving, and then Christmas is right around the corner.

THERAPIST: What feelings come up when you start to think about Christmas?

ELAINE: Christmas has never been a happy time for me.

THERAPIST: What was last Christmas like for you?

ELAINE: Last year, I drove to Washington, D.C., to spend some time with my father. It didn't go very well. Since my mother died a couple of years ago, he's been a mess. He drank too much the entire visit. Oh, I don't want to go into the details right now, but it was a disaster.

THERAPIST: A disaster?

ELAINE: Completely. But being alone is worse.

THERAPIST: And now the unexpected news that you might lose a class you love to teach must certainly add to this distress.

ELAINE: Yes. You can see why I am feeling so depressed.

THERAPIST: Yes, I hope we can talk more about both topics, but it's beginning to make sense to me why yesterday was such a difficult day for you. You were facing two very upsetting situations, just when you were beginning to feel a tiny bit better.

ELAINE: But maybe it is a medication issue.

THERAPIST: Well, let's take a little time to review the symptoms that the paroxetine should improve. Before yesterday, how were you sleeping and eating?

ELAINE: Fine, both had improved. But, like I said, the last 24 hours have been unbearable.

THERAPIST: Have your energy and concentration improved at all since being on the paroxetine the last few weeks?

ELAINE: Before yesterday, I was doing much better overall.

THERAPIST: Before we started the medication, you would think about dying or hurting yourself but didn't have any intention to act on it. How is that now?

ELAINE: It had improved until yesterday. Now, I am thinking about jumping out of the window again, but again, it's just a thought. I don't plan on acting on it.

But it bothers me that it even crosses my mind. I hadn't thought about it for a couple of weeks.

THERAPIST: How do you understand the fact that you were feeling so much better before yesterday?

ELAINE: I don't know. Maybe the medicine just stopped working. I also know the lunch discussion upset me, as you mentioned.

THERAPIST: I think you are right that yesterday was difficult. The news about the potential changes in the English department is very upsetting. It doesn't help that the holidays are just around the corner. I wonder if the combination might make it difficult for a while.

Overall, I think the medication is starting to help alleviate your neurovegetative symptoms of depression. But the medicine doesn't prevent a person from feeling sorrow or pain about troubling experiences.

ELAINE: You think the medicine is working, but yesterday was so bad because of my worries?

THERAPIST: It's certainly a possibility. Yesterday sounds like it was a very upsetting day. The disheartening news caused some increase in your symptoms. To me, this doesn't mean that you necessarily need more medication, but that we need to talk more about your concerns regarding job stress and the holidays and how best to deal with them.

ELAINE: You can't just give me a pill to feel better?

THERAPIST: That's a natural wish, but the paroxetine won't protect you from feeling upset about your class or about Christmas. It makes sense that you have strong feelings about both of these issues.

Increasing the medicine might prove necessary in the future, but right now, I think we need to concentrate on the situations that are causing you quite a lot of pain. (*Pauses.*)

ELAINE: (*Sniffles.*) Yes, maybe it will be helpful to talk more about this. Usually I try to ignore how I feel, because it is so uncomfortable to talk about this stuff.

THERAPIST: So not only are the feelings very difficult, you have been very alone with them as well.

ELAINE: Yes.

Elaine's concern is a common point of confusion for patients who have just started taking medication. While a medication increase is indicated if neurovegetative symptoms are unrelenting, an increase in symptoms in response to a life stress is usually temporary. Psychotherapy is the indicated treatment for these intermittent emotional crises.

It is worth reconsidering whether Elaine might benefit from a higher dose of the medication if her impaired sleep, appetite, or suicidal ideation worsen in the ensuing days or weeks.

DIVIDING THE CARE

In many instances, it can be clinically necessary and/or beneficial to split a patient's psychotherapy and psychopharmacological care between two providers. The most common treatment split occurs when a patient starts psychotherapy with a nonmedical therapist and medication becomes necessary. It is almost always best for the patient to continue psychotherapy with her therapist and to obtain medication from a psychopharmacologist.

Sometimes medical issues impede the progress of a psychotherapy. A patient who intensely focuses on medication concerns with a prescribing psychotherapist rather than observing how emotional stressors impact mood may do better with two clinicians. In addition, if a patient has very labile emotions, such as an individual with borderline personality traits who experiences volatile mood swings, or a patient with rapidly cycling or mixed bipolar disorder, the appropriate medication regimen may be complicated and may require frequent modification. If the frequent focus on psychopharmacological issues starts to distract from the psychotherapy, dividing care may allow both treatments the time they deserve.

THE PATIENT WHO WOULD BENEFIT
FROM MEDICATIONS BUT DOESN'T
CONSIDER THEM A TREATMENT OPTION

Sometimes, even when a patient is not taking any psychotropics, the issue of medications plays an important and recurring role within a psychotherapy. I have encountered this situation when a patient repeatedly refuses to start or to complete a medication trial even though she is clearly suffering from symptoms that medications could alleviate. Often, such patients believe that taking medications is a sign of character weakness or that medications are chemical toxins that will cause multiple unbearable side effects. In either case, a psychotropic medication trial may be doomed from the get-go.

If the therapist becomes too invested in a patient's decision to take medication, both individuals can become severely frustrated. I've found that it is most therapeutic to view the patient's refusal of medications as another psychodynamic topic that deserves revisiting every once in a while. With this tack, the patient doesn't feel pressured, and often, over time (although it may be months or even years), the patient will reconsider medications as an option if her symptoms do not improve with psychotherapy alone. Example 13.5 illustrates how I might discuss this issue with Elaine if she completely refused a medication trial despite her barrage of severe depressive symptoms.

EXAMPLE 13.5

Discussing medication as an option for a patient who refuses psychopharmacological treatment although she would clearly benefit from it

ELAINE: Dr. Bender, my condition hasn't improved over the last 6 months, even though we have been meeting twice a week. It's become unbearable. What do we do now?

THERAPIST: I think it is time to talk again about a trial of an antidepressant to help you with these symptoms. The symptoms you are describing to me are consistent with an illness called major depression which can be extremely debilitating—as you can see. With medication developed specifically to treat depression, over 2–4 weeks there can be some improvement in sleep, appetite, interest and even in hopelessness and suicidality.

ELAINE: Oh, you know that I am not interested in medications. I've seen friends go crazy on psychiatric drugs. It's not a viable option for me.

THERAPIST: What did you experience with your friends?

ELAINE: Well, one of them was recently diagnosed with manic–depressive illness, but they didn't know this when they gave her medication for depression. After taking the pill for a week, she was unable to sleep. Over the next few days, she started hearing voices. She had to be hospitalized.

I'm not interested in going through that.

THERAPIST: It's natural that you wouldn't want that. It is true that a person with manic depressive illness can have this reversible but very scary reaction to an antidepressant, but we have no evidence that you have this illness. For the vast majority of people, antidepressants are well-tolerated and extremely helpful.

ELAINE: I don't care. I don't want to put any new mind-altering medication in my body.

THERAPIST: Of course, that is your decision, but I hope that we can continue to discuss this over time.

ELAINE: You can discuss whatever you want, but my mind is made up.

THERAPIST: (*Nods, and waits to hear Elaine's next association.*)

ELAINE: I just hate feeling so alone every night.

THERAPIST: I can understand how it might feel particularly painful to feel alone while you are already feeling so vulnerable. What is a typical evening like for you?

ELAINE: Well, . . .

One Month Later

ELAINE: Dr. Bender, I'm still feeling like I can barely make it to work every day.

THERAPIST: Let's review some of the symptoms you were struggling with previously. How well are you sleeping and eating? How is your energy?

ELAINE: My appetite is a tad better, but I still have trouble sleeping every night, and my energy has been gone for months.

THERAPIST: How about the hopelessness and suicidality? Have those feelings increased, decreased, or stayed the same?

ELAINE: Well, I'm not thinking about suicide as much, but I am still pretty hopeless.

THERAPIST: You really are suffering. I feel stuck in a certain way, because I believe a trial of an antidepressant could be so helpful for you, but you have not even wanted to discuss it. Could we revisit the issue?

ELAINE: No! It's not an option for me.

THERAPIST: The depression is taking a toll on your body over time with just the decreased sleep. Would you be willing to discuss the option of a sleeping medication at least to help you through these difficult nights?

ELAINE: I'll have to think about that, but right now I am not interested in taking anything.

THERAPIST: You have very strong feelings about this issue.

ELAINE: Yes, I do.

THERAPIST: Can you tell me more why medications don't seem like a viable option to you?

ELAINE: If I improve, I want it to be because I helped myself, not because I popped a pill.

THERAPIST: Taking a pill makes you feel like the improvement isn't truly earned, that it isn't really yours?

ELAINE: I guess that's true. That is how I feel.

THERAPIST: There appears to be a conflict. You want to feel better but you reject some help that I'm offering. This method has left you isolated, lonely, and with an unrelenting depression. Perhaps we can try to understand together why some kinds of help are acceptable and other are not.

In Example 13.5, I illustrate some strategies that may be helpful for a patient who refuses to consider medication. First, I try to remain open and interested in Elaine's opinion and not to become too invested in the idea that she needs to start medications immediately. Therapy alone can be a great support to a patient. Increased resolution of one's underlying conflicts can sometimes diminish neurovegetative symptoms.

The next time Elaine openly complains about her distressing symptoms, I reopen the issue of medication. My understanding of Elaine's concerns is deepened as we continue to discuss the topic. Repeating this pattern, a review of the medication issue and a clarification of her concerns, might help Elaine reevaluate her stance over time. This scenario also illustrates how resistance to medication can reveal a profound psychodynamic conflict: aversion to help on one side and loneliness on the other.

If a patient refuses to take medications and continues to suffer from symptoms that could be easily targeted by psychotropics, our clinical power and ability to intervene effectively is limited. As psychotherapists, whether or not we prescribe, our job is to help patients to understand their condition and to provide an environment in which recovery and psychological growth can take place. Whether the patient takes advantage of this opportunity is ultimately up to him or her. Meanwhile, our task is to understand the process and to help the patient as much as she will permit.

Key words: benefits, citalopram, diagnosis, fantasies, fluoxetine, informed consent, integrative therapy, licensure, medicine, neurochemistry, neuropsychiatry, neurotransmitters, neurovegetative symptoms, paroxetine, prescribing practices, psychoeducation, psychopharmacology, psychotherapy, psychotropic, resistance, risks, selective serotonin reuptake inhibitors (SSRIs), sertraline, therapeutic alliance, therapeutic contract

Part IV
Therapeutic Dilemmas

14

Management of Impasses

An impasse is a pause in the progress of a psychotherapy. The therapist must gain an understanding of the dynamics of the impasse through careful listening, gentle inquiry, and empathic responsiveness. A resolution may be reached by means of clarifications and interpretations.

When I started training, I found the process of psychotherapy both fascinating and anxiety-provoking. When faced with a therapeutic dilemma I hadn't encountered before, I coped with my nervousness by adopting a "fix-it" attitude. I dispensed lots of advice and direct guidance. "Coulds" and "shoulds" would start to dominate my sentences. As Sallie's therapist, I might advise her to confront her mother directly about her career concerns. She should find a new friend to replace Gwen. She could join the school paper. And on and on.

Although my intentions were good, my instructive approach definitely impeded my patients' therapeutic progress. It was rare that a patient would follow my advice (If it were that easy, why would they be seeing me in the first place?), and sometimes the therapeutic alliance seemed to suffer after one of my overzealous interventions. As I started to observe my behavior more closely, I tried to understand which situations triggered my directive stance.

With some supervisory guidance, I learned that I became more preachy whenever I felt the therapy was at a standstill. My anxiety increased as I listened to a patient share a few of her concerns repeatedly without increased understanding or emotional relief. As a beginner, I didn't know that most therapies pass through some slow-moving stages. Instead, I attributed the lack of progress to my inexperience, and I reacted by dispensing more and more advice.

Over time, I've learned a number of alternative techniques that help a therapist and patient weather a therapeutic impasse. In this chapter, we'll illustrate several ways to respond to a slow-down in Sallie's treatment, modeling effective and ineffective techniques.

First, let's review how Sallie's therapy has progressed so far. Sallie came to therapy seeking help after her breakup with her boyfriend, Charlie. However, with time, as revealed in the last few chapters, it is increasingly evident that her troubles are more complicated than they had seemed.

While reviewing her family history, Sallie disclosed that her relationships with her mother and her brother, Tom, are sometimes difficult. Tom has suffered from a chronic disease for years, and Sallie has alluded (in Example 10.1) to Tom's medical needs monopolizing their mother's attention.

On the college front, once Sallie recovered from the acute stress of her breakup with Charlie, most of the therapy has focused on her relationship with her bossy friend, Gwen. It's psychologically interesting that Sallie has invested so much time and energy into this nonsupportive friendship. Simultaneously, Sallie continues her studies in economics, the major her mother chose for her, even though Sallie's heart isn't invested in the subject.

Sallie spends multiple sessions discussing these issues repetitively. Gwen is often mean, and Sallie is intensely sensitive to every rebuff. When Tom is ill, Sallie's mother is less available emotionally. Even though Sallie doesn't enjoy her current choice of study, economics, she revels in her mother's attention when they discuss her professional future.

During Examples 14.1 and 14.2, Sallie talks about these topics once again. Although beginning therapists may rely on responses like those modeled in Example 14.1, these tactics are unlikely to advance a treatment and may even undermine the therapeutic alliance.

EXAMPLE 14.1

The therapist employs ineffective tactics in response to an impasse in the treatment

Sallie is talking about her studies in economics as well as her continuing difficulties with her friendship with Gwen.

SALLIE: Well, I don't have anything that new to say today, Dr. Bender. I hate Economics 103. Hate it, hate it, hate it! And I thought it couldn't get worse after the intro courses. Well, I was wrong. Another great semester to look forward to, I guess. (*sarcastically*) Lucky me.

THERAPIST: What is it that you hate about Economics 103?

[*I choose the direction of the session right away, instead of helping Sallie to associate freely for the first 10–15 minutes of our meeting.*]

SALLIE: It's just so boring. I know if I study the information, I'll do fine, but I just don't like it.

THERAPIST: [*I feel frustrated because Sallie has been unhappy with her studies for months now, but never seems to do anything about it.*] Well, you could change majors. Maybe that would help. [*I give advice in hope of promoting psychological change.*]

SALLIE: Oh, that's not an option at all. I need to be an economics major. It's a done deal.

THERAPIST: What if you make list of all the aspects of economics that you like and dislike and we could review it together? [*I assign a cognitive task.*]

SALLIE: Okay, I guess I could do that.

THERAPIST: So, what about your other classes? How are they? [*I feel unsure how to help Sallie resolve these issues she talks about every week, so I redirect the conversation in an attempt to talk about a new topic.*]

SALLIE: Well, I love my journalism class. I love writing the assignment articles.

THERAPIST: Maybe you should join the school paper. [*I recommend action, moving away from affect. I'm relying heavily on "should" and "could," a sign that I am feeling increasingly unsure how to help Sallie.*]

SALLIE: Oh, I'm not that serious about it. It's a class for fun. Journalists don't make much money. It's not a viable future option for me. But I would like to tell you more about my latest tiff with Gwen.

Next Session

THERAPIST: So, did you make out your sheet listing the pros and cons of studying economics?

SALLIE: Oh, I didn't. I totally forgot to do it. My Mom was excited to hear about my latest assignments, so I spent a lot of time talking to her this week. She was really supportive, especially after Gwen was such a turd.

THERAPIST: [*I minimize Sallie's distress out of my own frustration.*] Your friendship with Gwen hits some trouble spots now and then, but you look like you are handling it well.

SALLIE: Well, maybe I look okay, but I feel like crap. I know I should be looking for new friends, and I've tried to spend less time with Gwen. It's hard though. When she's nice to me, I don't want to spend time with anyone else.

I don't get it. Sometimes she's amazing and tells me that I am the best friend she has ever had, and other times, she's just mean. I don't know how she'll act one minute to the next.

THERAPIST: It must be a great stress to be with a friend that makes you feel like crap. Why don't you find some new friends who treat you well? [*I stop minimizing, but recommend action instead in an attempt to help.*]

SALLIE: How can you say that? Even though the friendship is sort of up and down, I still think of Gwen as my best friend. She's all I have, except for you, and I pay you to listen to me.

THERAPIST: You have been struggling with this for a while now. Do you ever imagine your relationship with Gwen improving?

SALLIE: (*Tears arise.*) I don't know. I'm just scared to do anything.

THERAPIST: I understand that you are scared, but you'll keep suffering unless you change something about this situation! Do you have any idea why you stick with her?

SALLIE: Because she is special to me. That's all I know.

THERAPIST: Can you say anything else about it? Think hard. [*I push for cognitive understanding on an emotional topic. This tactic doesn't promote Sallie's understanding of her actions.*]

SALLIE: No. I don't want to talk about this anymore. Can we talk about something else?

THERAPIST: [*I confront the resistance head on.*] If you never talk about this, how can the situation ever improve?

SALLIE: Just forget it. I know it doesn't make sense, but Gwen is special to me, even though the friendship is so complicated. I wish you could understand that. Maybe this therapy just isn't working.

THERAPIST: I understand more than you think. For some reason, you stick with Gwen despite the fact that she treats you so poorly. She holds a lot of power over you, just like your mother does. [*My therapeutic hypothesis: Gwen doesn't feel replaceable because she is an emotional stand-in for someone unique in Sallie's life—probably her mother. Maybe that's why she sticks with a friend who continually hurts her feelings.*]

SALLIE: (*more tears*) I don't understand what you are getting at. Gwen isn't anything like my mother. But she is my best friend. Even if she doesn't treat me well lately, I can't just give up on a friendship that I have had for years.

Sallie misses the next session and doesn't call or cancel.

My anxiety and sense of helplessness fuel my ineffective directive approach illustrated in Example 14.1. If anything, Sallie becomes more protective of her emotional status quo as I push for her to change.

At the beginning of the example, I direct the content of the session prematurely rather than encouraging Sallie to associate more freely. Next, I try to instigate change by suggesting how to "fix" Sallie's situation ("Well, you could change majors.") and organizing her thinking by assigning cognitive homework (listing the pros and cons of an economics major). While a cognitive approach can be extremely useful to calm and to redirect a patient who is drowning in affect, it is not the best strategy for Sallie who needs more help getting in touch with her emotions.

Next, I redirect the topic of conversation rather than following Sallie's lead ("What about your other classes?"), and minimize Sallie's ongoing concerns about Gwen. ("Your friendship with Gwen hits some trouble spots now and then. You look like you are handling it well.") Finally, as my frustration mounts, I aggressively confront Sallie's resistance and interpret her behavior in an unempathic manner. ("Gwen holds a lot of power over you, just like your mother does.")

These expressions of my internal frustration are examples of countertransference enactments. These particular enactments involve complementary identification: Sallie's behavior evokes a domineering attitude in me that is similar to the mind-set of Gwen and of Sallie's mother. (For more about countertransference, see Chapter 16).

Sallie reacts as many patients might. Her views of Gwen become more entrenched rather than more flexible. From her perspective, this makes emotional sense. If it has always been difficult for Sallie to examine her relationship with Gwen, a bulldozing confrontation will only increase her resistance. Sallie manifests her intensified resistance by avoiding the next session.

I would have been more effective if I had helped Sallie discover her inner barriers to change instead of providing instruction. As Sallie's self-awareness slowly increased, she might find it easier to expand the limited range of life choices she currently allows herself.

Example 14.2 replays the previous example and employs a number of tactics that may be more conducive to progress when therapy reaches an impasse.

EXAMPLE 14.2

The therapist employs effective responses to the therapeutic impasse

SALLIE: Well, I don't have anything that new to say today, Dr. Bender. I hate Economics 103. Lucky me.

THERAPIST: (*Nods.*) [*I am trying not to intervene too early in the session, so I can hear how Sallie's concerns develop.*]

SALLIE: I guess I should be more interested in the class and not complain. I heard that graduating business majors have their choice of jobs. I have to keep reminding myself of this when I start to feel upset about my classes.

THERAPIST: (*Nods again.*) [*While I am purposely staying quiet to allow Sallie to talk freely and to reveal new material, I am staying emotionally involved in the conversation nonverbally through body language and frequent eye contact.*]

SALLIE: (*Continues to associate freely.*) Sometimes I wonder what it will be like to be in the business world after graduation. I guess it will be fine.

THERAPIST: What do you imagine it will be like?

SALLIE: I don't know. Maybe a little bit boring. I'm sure I'll grow to love it though.

THERAPIST: [*I try to learn more details that are affect-laden. Why does Sallie chose to study a subject that she doesn't really like? I wonder whether emotional forces that she is unaware of prevent her from changing majors.*] Can you tell me any more about what you imagine it will be like after graduation?

SALLIE: I'm sure it will be fine. It has to be.

THERAPIST: It has to be? What do you mean? [*I repeat a sentence that doesn't make logical sense but seems to have a lot of emotion beneath it.*]

SALLIE: I need to get some work experience after I graduate and then go on to get my MBA. It's basically already decided.

THERAPIST: How was it decided?

SALLIE: It's just the way it is. Umm, I don't really feel that comfortable talking about this, Dr. Bender.

THERAPIST: It doesn't feel like a subject that you want to explore more deeply?

SALLIE: Right. There is no use. Why talk about something that has already been decided?

THERAPIST: Can you explain to me how it was decided? [*I try one more time to help Sallie investigate her decision in more depth.*]

SALLIE: Well, I've told you how my mother has had a lot of influence on my career decisions. She wants to make sure I don't make the same mistakes she did.

THERAPIST: What were those?

SALLIE: I don't know. She always talks about her wish to open her own business some day, but in the next sentence, she'll say how glad she is to have a flexible job so she can take care of her children. Tom's illness underlined this point. (*looks away*)

Mom was an amazing student in college. But then she got married and had us in her early 20s, so she didn't pursue her career before we were born. In fact, she only started working in real estate a few years ago. When we were little, she was at home full time. I loved the time with her, but I wonder if she missed out on some of her dreams.

Maybe she's a little sad that she never had the chance to pursue her ideal career. She'd never say that, but it's easy to infer it by the way she talks. Sometimes, I wonder whether she'd make different choices if she could do it over.

THERAPIST: If she could do it over, what choice do you think she'd make this time?

SALLIE: I think she'd really go for it when she was younger. I don't know how she'd resolve the work/children issue, but I think she would be a great corporate executive. I can imagine her as the head of a startup company. She's a very smart woman.

Maybe it helps her to cheer me on instead. She always tells me that it's really important that I choose a profession that will make me an empowered woman who is financially independent. Business school seemed the best way to go about it. We decided that together.

THERAPIST: How did you and your mother come to this decision? [*I follow the emerging theme to gain a deeper understanding of the issue.*

I also think silently about the fact that Sallie's directive approach toward Charlie was very similar to her mother's approach with her.]

SALLIE: Well, even before I started college, my mother started talking to me about how to plan a profitable career. I don't need to be rich, but I want to be able to support myself easily and to pursue leadership roles. My mother says these are the two key factors to look for in a career.

How many daughters have mothers that take the time to discuss this stuff with them? I'm lucky, I think.

She thinks business, law, or medical school are the three best choices. Law and medicine aren't options for me. I've never been interested in law at all, and I'm so squeamish that I had trouble with dissections in high school biology. I couldn't handle medical school. Business school leaves me a lot of choices. It's what we've decided I should do.

So being upset about my classes is a waste of time. I don't know why I even bother complaining about it in here.

THERAPIST: How is it a waste of time?

SALLIE: Well, if it's a done deal, why am I struggling against it?

THERAPIST: Part of our work together involves recognizing your feelings, and sometimes feelings and thoughts are in conflict. What would it feel like to consider a major other than economics and a future career in something other than business? [*a strategic question that asks Sallie about her feelings, but doesn't suggest that she act any differently*]

SALLIE: I don't know. I just don't.

THERAPIST: (*Nods empathically.*)

SALLIE: I don't know. I guess I'd feel overwhelmed if I started thinking about changing the plan.

THERAPIST: What would feel overwhelming about it?

SALLIE: Umm, it just feels wrong. I don't really want to talk about it.

THERAPIST: It gives me a sense of how wrong it must feel if even thinking about other options feels overwhelming. But thinking isn't the same as acting. What do you imagine your mother would feel if she thought you had any misgivings about your major?

SALLIE: I think she'd be mad. College is a privilege, not a right. That's what she says to me all the time, and I appreciate my parents' support. I don't want to squander my studies on a major that doesn't have any potential.

THERAPIST: Which majors don't have potential?

SALLIE: I don't know. I guess journalism is the one I am thinking about specifically. If I knew I would be successful at it, I might major in journalism.
But I don't really like to talk about this.

THERAPIST: What does it feel like to talk about this?

SALLIE: I feel nervous. Uneasy.

THERAPIST: Where do you feel it in your body? [*I help Sallie expand on her feelings by describing her emotions in terms of other senses.*]

SALLIE: My stomach, I guess.

THERAPIST: How would you describe it?

SALLIE: I feel nauseous. Queasy.

THERAPIST: It's clearly a tender topic. Sometimes it can be easier to learn more about a troubling subject by using imagery. When you talk about this does any particular image come to mind?

SALLIE: I feel like a little mole and I want to burrow back into my hole.

THERAPIST: It's an interesting image. Can you tell me any more about the mole?

SALLIE: I don't know. I just feel confused, and it's easier to hide out in a little cave.

THERAPIST: Are you alone down there?

SALLIE: Oh yes, definitely. There's not enough room down here for anyone else.

THERAPIST: What does it feel like to be alone?

SALLIE: Okay actually. It's safer than having to worry about any other moles. (*Grins as she is involved in the imagery and metaphor.*)

THERAPIST: (*Smiles back.*) Hmmm, what would be your worry if there were any other moles?

SALLIE: I'm not sure, but I like having my own space. I don't have to worry about anyone else, and I feel safe. I don't feel squished, and I don't have to worry that the other mole would try to take over. It's all mine.

THERAPIST: Sharing is dangerous because the person might not just share but also take over?

SALLIE: Yeah, now that you mention it, I do feel like that.

THERAPIST: The images are very powerful. Do they feel familiar to you?

SALLIE: Sort of. . . .

THERAPIST: (*Raises eyebrows.*) [*nonverbal message: "Please go on."*]

SALLIE: Ummm, when I really think about it, I feel this way fairly often.

THERAPIST: Can you tell me more?

SALLIE: Well, first at school, I feel it with Gwen. She takes over when she bosses me around. I know it sounds stupid, but I worry she will also take away my other friends. Does that sound stupid?

THERAPIST: It sounds fearful, not stupid. Have you felt this way in any other places?

SALLIE: I sometimes feel this on trips home. Maybe sometimes with my brother.

THERAPIST: (*Nods.*)

SALLIE: Don't get me wrong. Tom's a great person. When he's healthy he's unstoppable. He's popular, handsome, and smart. I'm just not as interesting or talented as he is. When he's in a room, people are drawn to him. That doesn't happen to me. And when he's sick, people are drawn to him because he's ill, and he needs special care.

   I understand that. I'm lucky to be healthy. I'm not jealous of that type of attention.

   I don't know. I like the idea of having a safe place to hide out that I wouldn't need to share with anyone. (*Smiles.*)

THERAPIST: Climbing down into your hole to stay safe and protect your space?

SALLIE: Yes. Sometimes, I even resent the fact that Tom's illness intrudes into my therapy hour. Isn't that horrible! I just like having you all to myself. I want to talk about me, not him.

   Anyway, when Tom is well, he's better at most things than I am. I'm good at sports; he's great. I'm okay at math; it's his favorite subject.

THERAPIST: Talking about him feels like you have to share me with him?

SALLIE: In a certain way, it really does.

THERAPIST: Let's look at the associations here. Maybe you have an idea how to put them together. At first you talked about your mother and about her concern about your choice of study. Your next association and image involved the mole, and then Tom, and not wanting to share anything or anyone with him. Do the two images seem related to you in any way? [*I have an idea how they might be related, but it would be much more effective and informative if Sallie were able to tie the two together.*]

SALLIE: Well, maybe a little bit. Tom has never had to work for my Mom's attention. Even before he was sick, he was the more charismatic kid. He couldn't help it, and my Mom and him always seemed to have a special bond. I wasn't really jealous. Well, maybe just a little bit.

But then, when he got sick, all bets were off. He needed Mom more, and she was always there for him. I shouldn't be jealous of that. He was suffering. I'm glad she paid so much attention to him.

But, I've got one thing on Tom. I'm the only daughter, and Mom enjoys being my mentor. She's always taken a special interest in my studies. It's one area that I have Tom licked. I hope you can understand why I wouldn't want to change anything. Mom and I bond over this stuff at school.

THERAPIST: That makes a lot of sense. I can understand that you would want to protect this special bond with your Mom.

SALLIE: I know, but for some reason, I still don't feel good about economics.

THERAPIST: That is really the dilemma. Your choice of classes continues to bother you for reasons we don't fully understand at this point, but even discussing it feels uncomfortable, both emotionally and physically. [*I verbalize Sallie's dilemma without any expectation that she will act any differently.*]

SALLIE: That's true. So what do I do?

THERAPIST: I think we need to search for greater understanding of the problem.

SALLIE: Maybe so, but right now, I'd rather move on and tell you about Gwen.

THERAPIST: Sure. Perhaps we can talk more about your classes and career goals another time. [*While I follow Sallie's lead in changing the subject, I make a comment about the unfinished business.*]

Example 14.2 illustrates a number of effective procedures that may help a treatment evolve beyond the therapeutic impasse. All the tactics attempt to look at the same emotional material through a different lens in order to understand old concerns in a new way.

At the beginning of the session, I remain relatively quiet to facilitate Sallie's associations, rather than to direct them prematurely. This approach can be very helpful to many patients who use the first 10–15 minutes of a session to "warm up" toward a troubling topic. Even though I don't talk much, my silence is an amiable one. While I avoid any comments that might interfere with the gradual emergence of new material, I use nonverbal cues to portray my interest.

If Sallie seemed uncomfortable with this approach, I might ask her to describe how she experiences the silence. ("As we sit here together, I am wondering what this silence is like for you?") Learning how Sallie interprets my less active approach may reveal some useful information.

As the session evolves, I ask Sallie a number of detailed questions about her school concerns rather than assuming that we had exhausted this recurring topic. Her replies slowly reveal how her choice to study economics is tied to an understandable desire for her mother's attention and approval. Before Sallie will be ready to make any significant changes in her career path, we need to appreciate her conflicting wishes and fears in more detail.

As illustrated in Example 14.1, direct confrontation in this situation may increase her resistance. In fact, if I insisted that Sallie choose an alternative career path, I would be acting like her mother by directing Sallie's life according to my priorities.

Instead, I acknowledge and respect Sallie's resistance by gently asking what it would feel like if she didn't experience these internal limitations. The question is worded very carefully. I don't recommend that Sallie change her perspective or act any differently. ("What would it feel like to consider a major other than economics and a future career in something other than business?")

We discuss Sallie's concerns in displacement, first focusing on where she feels her distress in her body and then helping Sallie develop her image of herself as a shy mole. Sallie mentions that her space will not feel protected if it is shared. In response to open-ended questions, she is able to relate her metaphor of the mole to her feelings about her brother and mother.

Although Sallie is able to talk about her fantasy in detail, these strategies may be useful even if her image had been less well-defined. If Sallie's image were more murky, ("I just see a grey fog"). I might ask more questions to develop the image ("Does this remind you of anything in particular?" or "What might be hidden in the fog?"). If I am open to this creative venture, she is likely to follow. For a more aurally inclined patient, I might ask, "Does this make you think of any type of music or sound?" With an action-oriented patient, I may ask about impulses: "When you talk about this, do you feel an impulse to do something?" Many an emotion that cannot be tapped verbally can be explored through a creative displacement or an affective equivalent.

At a certain point, I ask Sallie if she sees any connection between her mole image and her concerns about Tom and her mother. She revisits her emotional dilemma: In order to stay close to her mother, she doesn't want to assert an independent career choice. I empathize with her concerns, ("That makes a lot of sense. I can understand that you would want to protect this special bond with your Mom.") and acknowledge the emotional complexity of the issue ("Your choice of classes continues to bother you for reasons we don't fully understand at this point, but even discussing it feels uncomfortable, both emotionally and physically.").

Soon after, Sallie changes the topic back to Gwen. It isn't unusual for a patient to have a limited tolerance for an emotionally intense subject. In response, I note that it would be useful for us to continue our discussion about Tom and her mother in the future, and then follow her lead to the next topic.

INTERPRETATIONS AND CLARIFICATIONS

In addition to careful listening, gentle open-ended questions, and non-verbal encouragements, interpretations and clarifications can advance a psychotherapy. Interpretations are comments that link the patient's past experiences with her present, for example, "Your boss's self-centered approach is so difficult for you to tolerate because he reminds you of your father." Clarifications are explanatory interventions that do not necessarily include a historical or developmental perspective. (In Example 14.2, my question "Sharing is dangerous because the person might not just share but also take over?" is a clarification.) Both of these interventions help the patient to think, to feel, and to talk about very sensitive subjects. They may be met by some resistance, the psychological defenses a person may use to protect herself from emotional distress.

When I started psychiatric training after a year of internal medicine replete with clear, objectively based diagnoses and algorithmic treatment plans, I imagined interpretations and clarifications as verbal procedures that could dissect emotional pain and immediately relieve distress. If I could manage to "explain" the patient's inner motivations, a sustained cure would follow. I felt confident that a healing interpretation existed for each patient. I just had no idea what it was or where to find it.

During my first few years as a psychotherapist, I tried to make this fantasy come true multiple times. Many hours were spent offering various epiphanies to my few psychotherapy patients, hoping beyond hope that I had hit the therapeutic jackpot. Needless to say, it never worked. Even if the patients were polite and acknowledged my attempt to "solve" their problems, their conditions never seemed to improve after my psychological sermons.

I reevaluated my method after one patient disappeared for 3 months following one of my "enlightening" comments. In my haste to interpret her distress, she may have felt misunderstand and emotionally exposed. Finally, I realized that a psychotherapeutic cure cannot be distilled into one or two beard-stroking interpretations.

Although the wish for curative interpretation is certainly understandable, psychotherapy is a lengthy process without any easy answers. In fact, the therapist who can endure a problem's ambiguity and avoid pigeonholing the patient's experience does her patient a much greater service than the therapist who is overeager to reach a simplifying explanation.

The following examples will illustrate how overinterpretation or overclarification can flummox a treatment, while their careful use at the right time can promote understanding.

CLARIFICATIONS: MISUSE AND USE

Example 14.3 illustrates how a well-meaning beginner may misuse the art of clarification after hearing a patient's dream.

EXAMPLE 14.3

Premature and inaccurate clarifications

SALLIE: Dr. Bender, I had the weirdest dream last night. Can I tell you about it? I felt sort of shook up when I woke up this morning.

THERAPIST: Please, I'd like to hear about it. [*I'm excited and nervous to hear about the dream but feel some immediate pressure and responsibility to understand and to explain its underlying meaning during this session.*]

SALLIE: Well, okay. I remember swimming in a deep, dark river. It was warm and very comfortable, and I felt like a fish, which is funny because I'm not a very good swimmer. Instead of hands, I think I had some fins that glowed in the dark. It was so calm and peaceful; the river slowly crept along and I swam with the current. Then, I saw a cave. I crept inside of it, and it was really dark but I could make out this ledge on the side of the cave that had enough room for me to lie down. All of a sudden I got really tired and didn't feel strong enough to keep going, so I went to sleep on the ledge. And that's when I woke up, feeling upset. . . .

THERAPIST: [*I am excited that I have thought of a clarification, and I interrupt, happy that I have thought of something smart to say.*]

Somehow you needed to escape the river; it wasn't safe to continue swimming by yourself.

SALLIE: Huh?

THERAPIST: I am just struck by the fact that the cave served as an escape so you would no longer have to move forward alone in the river. As you are in school and growing in independence, it's scary. Sometimes you may want to find a cave that is safe to hide in.

SALLIE: Oh, is that what it meant?

THERAPIST: That is how I understand it, anyhow. [*I feel a bit proud and smug.*]

SALLIE: That's interesting. Umm, I wanted to make sure that I tell you what happened in school yesterday. Gwen has been up to her usual tricks.

THERAPIST: [*I nod but miss the fact that Sallie has chosen to change topics rather abruptly.*]

SALLIE: You know, I think Gwen might hate me! (*Starts to cry, which is unexpected by both of us.*)

THERAPIST: What happened?

SALLIE: I don't know. (*Chokes through sobs.*) She's ignored all of my calls this week. I don't know what I did wrong. I must have done something to cause this. I feel so guilty.

THERAPIST: [*I feel an urgent need to relieve Sallie's distress and jump to explain Sallie's behavior.*] You feel guilty so easily. As you gain independence, Gwen is shutting you out, and guilt is a much easier emotion than anger.

SALLIE: Oh, I don't feel angry at Gwen. She's my closest friend. (*Becomes silent for a few moments.*) I don't like to criticize her. I have a big economics test next week. It's on a ridiculous amount of material. I have no idea how I am going to prepare.

THERAPIST: Why the change in subject all of a sudden? Did I say something to upset you?

SALLIE: I don't know. I am just sick of talking about this stuff all the time. The situation with Gwen is really hard.

In Example 14.3, I try to make sense of the dream after hearing Sallie briefly outline it only one time. In my fantasy as a novice psychotherapist, this is Sallie's cue to say something like: "Eureka! I finally understand that I try to avoid making independent decisions because of a complicated dynamic with my parents that I can just now understand. Thank you so much. I know my life will be different now." Example 14.3 is more reality-based. Sallie's passive agreement is a common response to an overzealous therapeutic approach.

When Sallie changes the subject to discuss her ongoing difficulties with Gwen, I repeat my previous error and present another clarification of Sallie's behavior. ("Guilt is a much easier emotion than anger.") Two premature clarifications in a row reflect more on my internal state than the patient's. In this situation, it is a signal that I am probably feeling anxious, insecure about my psychotherapeutic skills, and frustrated about the patient's slow progress.

Even though I have good intentions when I try to resolve Sallie's difficulties, Sallie begins to cry after my comments. From her perspective, my intervention may have felt more like an emotional assault. Yet, when I ask her directly how she experienced our discussion, Sallie doesn't tell me how uncomfortable my comments made her feel. She blames her emotional distress on the situation with Gwen.

The more therapeutic approach is less flashy and more humble. Nowadays, if I think I understand something very quickly, I suspect that I probably don't understand it thoroughly, because most significant issues are multiply determined. When a patient first reports a dream or a difficult situation, I'll ask more questions and withhold my opinion. I'll also try to elicit associations to some of the more salient elements of the story. Basic queries such as "Let's try to understand this together. Can you tell me more about the dark cave? How does it feel to tell me about it?" serve me well, and help the patient disclose details that she hadn't been aware of before.

After hearing about a patient's dream, I may have a hypothesis regarding what it might reveal, but only further and deeper discussion with the patient will show whether I'm even in the right ballpark. In fact, I've found that it is rare that any dream or personal dilemma is fully understood during the session in which it is reported.

Example 14.4 illustrates how a therapist can use a dream as nourishing fodder for discussion without jumping to clarify its meaning.

EXAMPLE 14.4

Using a dream to clarify the goals of therapy

SALLIE: Dr. Bender, I had the weirdest dream last night. Can I tell you about it?

THERAPIST: Sure. (*waits patiently*)

Sallie presents the same dream as in Example 14.3.

THERAPIST: It's an interesting dream. Thank you for sharing it with me. Let's go through it again a bit more slowly. Can you tell me the beginning again?

SALLIE: Okay. First, I just remember swimming in this slow relaxing river. I was all alone, but I didn't feel lonely. I felt very adventurous instead of feeling scared. That is one of the weird parts because, like I said, I'm usually not that comfortable in the water.

THERAPIST: What else did you feel during the dream?

SALLIE: Well, in the beginning, I mainly felt free and not tied down at all. Before I climbed on the ledge, I felt that I could float or swim in the river forever. Something bad seemed to be missing.

THERAPIST: Something bad?

SALLIE: It seemed like I didn't feel bad about myself at all. Maybe that part of me that is always so self-critical was missing. I'm not sure.

THERAPIST: (Nods.)

SALLIE: Now as I listen to myself I feel annoyed. My dream was all about being free and feeling good about myself, but even as I talk about it, I hear this aggravating voice in my head making critical comments.

THERAPIST: What does the voice in your head say?

SALLIE: You know, it sounds like Gwen. I don't know. She'd think of some way to make me feel stupid about the dream. She's expert at that.

THERAPIST: A very critical voice in your head that sounds a little like Gwen. . . .

SALLIE: Yes, and in the dream, it didn't exist, at least while I was swimming, and that felt really great.

THERAPIST: I can understand that it would feel great to be free of self-criticism. What do you make of the river?

SALLIE: What do you mean?

THERAPIST: Well, did it remind you of any particular river or any particular place?

SALLIE: Umm, I don't know if the river in the dream was a river I have actually visited. The feeling of being free is a little bit familiar though. I used to feel this way during our family's summer trips to national parks. I don't think I've told you about this. We went to a different one almost every year. I always looked forward to it.

My mother always made a ceremony of taking off her watch as we drove through the park gates. She was more relaxed during these weeks than any other time of the year. We even went the summers that Tom wasn't feeling well. The trip might be a little shorter, but we always went.

As a kid, I loved those vacations. We all got along well, and it felt so relaxed and free. All the everyday stress was gone. It's hard to explain how good it was.

I always give money to the national parks every Christmas. I feel attached to them.

THERAPIST: It does sound like the parks have been a place of great freedom for you.

SALLIE: Yes, they were, but it doesn't make a lot of sense that my dream focused on swimming. I don't like to swim very much. I do like to hike, and we would do that together as a family, but I never manage to make time for it these days. There's actually a hiking club at school, but I haven't joined.

THERAPIST: Can you tell me what holds you back?

SALLIE: I don't know.

THERAPIST: [*As I continue to review the dream in my mind, I remember that Sallie also had a cave in her "mole" image from Example 14.2. I continue to be silent to see if Sallie starts talking again spontaneously. When she doesn't, I decide to ask a question.*] The cave, can you tell me how you felt in the cave?

SALLIE: I felt my old self creeping back while I was in the cave. I wasn't fearful during the first part of the dream, but in the second part it became very dark, and I started to get scared. I feel sort of stupid admitting it, but I actually get scared of the dark fairly often—when I'm awake, I mean.

THERAPIST: Can you tell me more about this fear of the dark? When do you feel it?

SALLIE: Mostly when I'm home alone, but I've also noticed that it definitely gets worse when I'm upset, like after a fight with Gwen.

THERAPIST: These observations are useful. They will help us understand the fear better. How do you act differently when you feel this fear?

SALLIE: I just get nervous and I'll check to see if the front door is locked. Sometimes, if I am really wigged out for some reason, I sleep with a light on. I just don't feel comfortable all by myself.

THERAPIST: And during the last part of the dream, you felt differently.

SALLIE: Yes, for a short while, I felt okay being by myself doing what I like to do, even if I wasn't the best at it.

THERAPIST: (*Nods empathically.*)

SALLIE: It's not like that in real life.

THERAPIST: The dream gave you a taste of what would it be like not to feel so afraid or self-critical while you are awake.

SALLIE: Yes, do you ever think I could feel less afraid?

THERAPIST: I think we are working on that together, even by talking about the dream. Over time, we may learn more about the dream and what it tells us about fear and freedom. With increased understanding, you might begin to feel more like you did as you swam down the river.

When Sallie slowly reports her dream the second time, I pay special attention to her emotional experience during each section. The type of exploration illustrated in Example 14.4 can also be used to facilitate any discussion, whether about a dream or about a difficult situation that the patient is struggling with during waking hours.

If I had more time to discuss the dream with Sallie, I would also ask her about the events of her day prior to the dream to see if that helps us understand more of the dream's meaning. Daytime experiences that find their way into a dream are known as the "day residue." Other questions such as "Does any particular part of the dream stand out to you? Are the feelings in the dream familiar to you? Where have you felt them before?" could further facilitate the discussion.

Once the discussion of the dream is finished, I'll take special notice of Sallie's next associations. In contrast to Example 14.3, I don't hazard a soundbite clarification that would prematurely connect all the pieces of the dream with the content of recent sessions.

Now and then my patient and I will discuss a dream in detail, and it still won't make any cohesive sense. While I often feel a pull to explain and to tie up the loose ends, the dream remains available for future exploration if I refuse to simplify it with a quick and dirty interpretation.

Sigmund Freud would sometimes spend weeks reviewing a dream with a patient. Because he was practicing psychoanalysis, he had the time to delve deeply into a dream to understand its underlying conflicts and its orgins. Once-a-week psychotherapy doesn't have this luxury, but dream material and the subsequent associations can be very valuable as inroads to new understanding.

The discussion in Example 14.4 does highlight some patterns in Sallie's thinking that would be useful to discuss some time in the future. It is noteworthy that Sallie is often fearful and is aware that this sensitivity makes life unnecessarily difficult. Meanwhile, as I've commented before,

Sallie is rarely openly angry in her dealings in life in general and with Gwen in particular. It's possible that the two are related.

Maybe Sallie's fearfulness has an unconscious purpose. A useful procedure in psychodynamic thinking is to look for the feeling opposite to the patient's conscious emotional experience. Perhaps Sallie's ubiquitous fear keeps her aggression in check. It is unclear why aggressive and angry impulses are unaccceptable to Sallie, but the recognition of this conflict may form the the seed of future insight.

INTERPRETATIONS

Interpretations differ from clarifications in that they tie together a patient's difficulties in the past and present in a meaningful way. To illustrate: Let's say I start to work in therapy with a 30-year-old woman we'll call Martha, who wants to discuss her ongoing difficulties with her critical and reproachful mother. As a child, she was intimidated by her mother's inflexible attitude. Her mother would scold or punish Martha if she didn't follow her instructions to the letter. In response, Martha learned to assert her independence covertly by withholding or delaying: classic passive–aggressive behaviors. While living at home and attending school, Martha wouldn't start her homework that was due Monday morning until late Sunday evening. Her mother would be aggravated by these delaying tactics, but Martha would always manage to complete most of the work on time. Although she might "forget" to relay an important message to her mother for a number of days, she would eventually share the information. Her mother became very annoyed by these behaviors and responded with an even more rigid attitude. By the time I met the patient, this cycle had been in place for years.

Martha might use similar withholding and delaying techniques in her current life or with me within the therapy. She may finish work projects at the last minute, irritating her coworkers, or repeatedly pay her therapy bill the week it would be considered overdue.

As the therapy progressed, I would try to help Martha connect her current actions in her adult life with her old ways of coping as a child. For this interpretation to be effective, we would need to discuss how this ineffective coping mechanism evolved and talk at length about Martha's understandable frustration and annoyance at her mother. Martha must feel that I understand the motivations for her past behavior before we can fully examine her present difficulties in relationships. Over time, as we maintain a nonjudgmental but curious approach, we may recognize together how Martha is using obsolete (and replaceable) coping mechanisms, possibly without conscious knowledge, in her current responsibilities and relationships.

Example 14.5 illustrates how an interpretation can link a patient's current difficulties with emotional struggles from her past.

EXAMPLE 14.5

The therapist interprets a patient's recurring difficulty with her friend

SALLIE: Ugh. Sometimes I hate Gwen, Dr. Bender, even though she is my best friend. Yesterday we had another fight. It ruins my whole evening when we battle.

THERAPIST: It is upsetting that these fights keep recurring with a friend who is so important to you. What happened?

SALLIE: Well, you know how I always let Gwen choose how we are going to spend our time together. After our last session, I figured it was time for a change, and last night I asked her to go with me to a campus reading. A senior had just returned from a year in Africa, and she wanted to talk and show slides about her experiences. I love travel and journalism—I might consider it as a profession if I knew I could make money at it—so I really wanted to go.

I was a little nervous asking Gwen to go with me, but I thought she might be interested. Well, anyway, she had already planned to go to a party in a nearby dorm, because a guy she likes was going to be there. I asked if we could go to the party after the talk, but she wouldn't compromise. It wouldn't have been a big deal if we could have just gone our separate ways for the evening. I suggested that idea, and she went completely ballistic.

THERAPIST: What did she say?

SALLIE: She said that I was a mediocre friend who couldn't be counted on, and joining her at the party after the talk just wouldn't cut it. If I really wanted to prove myself as a good dependable friend, I needed to come with her and help her meet this guy and skip the talk. Otherwise, her opinion of me had seriously declined, and I wasn't a true friend after all.

THERAPIST: How did it feel to you when she said this?

SALLIE: I felt horrible, so I skipped the talk and went to the party with her, and it was awful. It was so bizarre. Once she got her way, she was so grateful to have company. She said all these nice things to me.

This time it didn't make me feel any better. I kept reviewing the fight in my head last night, so I hardly slept at all.

Plus, remember I told you that sometimes I have trouble relaxing in the dark? Well, last night I kept the lights on all night. I still feel upset. (*Tears well up, and she reaches for a tissue.*)

THERAPIST: It sounds like a very upsetting evening. You have tried so hard to be a good friend to Gwen, but it is difficult when she doesn't allow you any leeway.

SALLIE: Yes! She really gets to me. But it was okay to have a separate idea and want to go to the talk, wasn't it?

THERAPIST: Of course it was, but the fact that you ask the question shows me that you aren't quite sure that it's okay for you to express a preference and still be a good friend.

SALLIE: Yeah. I do feel so unsure of myself with Gwen. Like I have to do things her way in order to make sure she still likes me.

THERAPIST: That is a great deal of pressure for you because it doesn't allow you to express any wishes you have that are different from Gwen's. How do you understand finding yourself in such a situation?

SALLIE: What do you mean?

THERAPIST: Well, have you ever experienced this type of relationship pressure with anyone else?

SALLIE: I don't know, maybe. I think I told you about my friends Claudia and Dawn. They were my best friends growing up. They were never as mean as Gwen, but sometimes they would be kinda bossy in the same way. But it's my fault, too. I just don't feel comfortable standing up for myself.

THERAPIST: Have you ever felt this way with anyone in your family?

SALLIE: Not that I can think of. Oh, I don't know.

THERAPIST: Well, I have an idea, but I don't know if it will feel right to you. Tell me what you feel about this.

SALLIE: Okay. What?

THERAPIST: Do you think the way you describe Gwen, Claudia, and Dawn sounds a little bit like the way you describe your mother?

SALLIE: What do you mean?

THERAPIST: Well, we've talked about your mother's influence on your career choice. On the one hand, it is a special bond that you two share, but your discussions don't leave room for alternate career choices.

SALLIE: And if my Mom got mad at me, I'd feel terrible.

THERAPIST: Terrible? Can you say more?

SALLIE: I just don't want to get in a fight with her. It's not worth it. I'm sure she knows what's best for me anyway. Economics isn't too bad.

THERAPIST: It is a difficult situation. I can understand why you would want to be able to talk to your mother more openly and share your ideas, but you don't want to risk her getting mad at you like Gwen did.

SALLIE: Right.

THERAPIST: The difficulty arises when you feel that you must ignore your own ideas and wishes to maintain an important relationship.

SALLIE: I know. I'm used to it though. My Mom and I get along the best when I do things her way.

THERAPIST: That may account for how the behavior evolved. When you were a child, it was easiest just to submerge your feelings and follow your mother's advice, but now that you are older, it is increasingly difficult because you have your own independent ideas.

In Example 14.5, I hazard an interpretation, tying Sallie's ongoing difficulties with Gwen with her fears of asserting herself with her mother. In fact, because Sallie has repeatedly chosen bossy friends who tell her what to do, she may be experiencing a "repetition compulsion." This term was coined by Freud and refers to situations in which a person tries to rework an old conflict through current relationships. It makes sense that Gwen may be an emotional stand-in for Sallie's mother. Gwen feels irreplaceable, like a mother, which is probably a reason why Sallie continues in the nonsupportive friendship.

I use several techniques to try to make the interpretation palatable to Sallie. Prior to the interpretation, I reinforce our therapeutic alliance by supporting Sallie's tentative move toward independence with Gwen. Then, before sharing my ideas, I first ask Sallie if she sees any similarities between her friendship with Gwen and any other important past relationships. After hearing Sallie's input, I strategically hedge the interpretation as a question. ("Do you think the way you describe Gwen, Claudia, and Dawn sounds a little bit like the way you describe your mother?") With this approach, the discussion will evolve around Sallie's agreement or disagreement with my ideas. Either way, our understanding of the topic deepens. Finally, as the conversation progresses, I explain my view of Sallie's behavior gently and with empathy for how it evolved over time.

Example 14.5 avoids a number of common pitfalls. The interpretation is not humiliating or condescending. It does not attempt to be a therapeutic epiphany. In fact, its power lies in the fact that it isn't a great surprise to Sallie. It reformulates information that Sallie has shared with me over time. It is only a slight stretch for Sallie to acquire the new perspective.

As Sallie's mother becomes the focus, Sallie might discover that she has, without conscious awareness, resented the control exerted by her mother's giving and withholding of attention. It's possible that much of that resentment was turned against herself in the forms of self-reproach, devaluing views of herself, impaired confidence, and unearned feelings of guilt. As she allows herself to express her hostile feelings in the safe arena of the therapy sessions rather than turning her anger inward, her self-assurance may increase.

Over time, she may also gain the courage to imagine talking to her mother, as one adult to another, about a career other than business. She may begin to conceive of the possibility of maintaining her mother's attention and care while pursuing her own interests and developing her own talents. If Sallie is game, mental imagery or rehearsals during the therapy sessions could help her prepare for a talk with her mother.

As these therapeutic developments emerge coincident with Sallie's improved ability to communicate, her relationship with her mother may improve. Even if they continue to disagree about Sallie's career opportunities, they may still feel closer if they are able to talk more openly and honestly. As Sallie's confidence increases and she realizes that ignoring her own feelings doesn't guarantee a fulfilling friendship, she might become more open with Gwen. If Gwen cannot tolerate mutuality, Sallie might start to search out new relationships.

While progress with such profound consequences may be triggered or catalyzed by well-timed interpretations, a large part of these changes will likely be mediated through the relationship between the patient and the therapist. We illustrate how these processes occur in the next two chapters.

Key words: affective equivalents, analysis of resistance, associations, clarification, confrontation, countertransference enactment, defense, dreams, imagery, impasse, insight, interpretation, passive-aggression, psychoanalysis, psychotherapy, repetition compulsion, resistance, sibling rivalry, working through

15

Empathic Lapses

An empathic lapse occurs when the therapist misunderstands the patient. If the lapse is not acknowledged by the therapist, the treatment may suffer. If the incident is recognized and discussed, the relationship and the treatment may be revitalized.

WHAT IS AN EMPATHIC LAPSE?

As a novice psychiatrist during the first months of my training, I'd fantasize about my future as the most empathic therapist of all time: a therapeutic superhero. Eventually, I would learn how to create psychological change in a single bound. I would cure long-standing emotional pain that had been resistant to all previous treatment. I would understand everything.

After I gained some clinical experience, my perspective on empathy underwent a fundamental change. Even if it were possible to do so, I'm no longer interested in becoming the most empathic therapist on record.

Misunderstandings, as unpleasant as they can be, offer unique therapeutic opportunities. Some patients avoid close relationships because of the "baggage" that accompanies them: a fear of being misunderstood and a fear of rejection. If I can model how to work through conflicts in a constructive manner while maintaining an emotional connection, my patient's trust in me and in her own capacity to bear intimacy will ultimately increase. Rather than aim for perfection, I now work toward relationship resiliency.

"Empathic failure" is the term used in the psychotherapeutic literature to describe an interaction in which the therapist misunderstands the patient. From our perspective, it's a harsh and inaccurate term. We've

259

employed the term "empathic lapse" as a replacement, promoting our view that these are not failures but valuable opportunities for discussion and learning.

A patient may respond to an empathic lapse in any number of ways. She might laugh and pretend it didn't happen, withdraw and cancel the next session, or cry openly and express how hurt she feels. I've found the angry patient the most challenging. It's comparatively easy to listen to a patient's rage regarding her family or friends, but it feels entirely different to have a patient's fury directed at me.

REACTING TO AN EMPATHIC LAPSE

The unprepared therapist may feel at a loss when faced with an angry patient after an empathic lapse. Example 15.1 illustrates how an inexperienced therapist might respond to this predicament.

EXAMPLE 15.1

An empathic lapse occurs between the patient and her therapist. The therapist responds by becoming defensive, focusing on the patient's past, and then trying to repair the misunderstanding too quickly

Midway into a Session with Sallie

SALLIE: I don't know, Dr. Bender. Sometimes I feel so independent, and other times I just want to curl up into a little ball and cry.

THERAPIST: So, sometimes you feel like an adult and other times you feel like a little girl?

SALLIE: (*Looks down at the floor and twists a tissue in her hands.*) I guess so.

Next Session

SALLIE: I don't have anything to say today.

THERAPIST: (*Nods, but does not say anything, hoping Sallie's associations will emerge naturally.*)

SALLIE: I am not a little girl! (*Blurts angrily.*)

THERAPIST: (*taken by surprise*) Huh?

SALLIE: Last session, you said this thing that just wasn't true. Remember when you said that I sometimes act like a little girl?

I don't know. Is that how you see me? I don't even know what to say to you anymore if that's the case.

I can't believe that I have been confiding in you for months, and you don't understand me at all.

THERAPIST: I said what?

SALLIE: Last session, I told you this very personal thing, and you called me a little girl.

You don't even remember? Whatever. Just forget it.

THERAPIST: I think this is important to talk about. As I remember it, I did not say you were a little girl. I said that sometimes you feel like a little girl.

SALLIE: It only feels worse to hear you say it again! You know, I had no idea you were this judgmental.

THERAPIST: I was not judgmental. I don't think I said that you were a little girl. I think you are remembering the interaction incorrectly.

SALLIE: Whatever . . . if you say so. . . . (*Breaks eye contact, and looks at the floor.*)

THERAPIST: It seems this really upset you.

SALLIE: Well, sort of. You usually understand what I say. I don't even know what to do now. I feel shot down.

THERAPIST: I must have reminded you of your mother. You have told me how alone you feel when your mother misunderstands something important about you and doesn't listen to your point of view.

SALLIE: Huh? (*Starts to cry.*) I don't want to talk about my mom. I wasn't even thinking about that.

THERAPIST: Can you tell me why you are crying?

SALLIE: Because you just don't get it.

THERAPIST: Am I reminding you of your mom right now?

SALLIE: No, you are not. I don't think you are like my mom at all. Just forget it.

THERAPIST: [*I don't know what to do, but I figure that validating Sallie's emotions can't hurt. I decide to change tactics.*] I can understand how hard it could feel to begin to trust me and then to feel "shot down."

SALLIE: I just don't understand what you meant if it wasn't a put-down.

THERAPIST: I definitely didn't mean to put you down. Let me think for a minute what I was trying to say.

I think I meant to say that you may have a part of you that sometimes feels like a little girl, while other parts of you are functioning like an independent adult. I am really sorry.

SALLIE: Well, I don't like to think about it in those terms. It seems derogatory to me.

THERAPIST: I didn't mean it in a derogatory way at all, but I can understand how painful it might be if that is how it sounded.

SALLIE: (*Looks uncomfortable.*) Yeah, yeah. Let's talk about something else.

Example 15.1 illustrates a number of common, understandable, but not very therapeutic tactics that a novice therapist might employ when faced with an unexpectedly angry patient after an empathic lapse. I start by defending my comment ("As I remember it, I did not say you were a little girl. I said that sometimes you feel like a little girl.") and Sallie reacts with agitation followed by withdrawal.

During my second defensive maneuver, I refer to Sallie's family dynamics to escape a direct discussion of my actions. ("I must have reminded you of your mother.") While my instinctual response to feeling ashamed isn't unusual, Sallie may experience the psychodynamic sidestepping as attacking. It isn't a therapeutically useful response.

By the end of the example, I become a bit more compassionate. I stop trying to argue Sallie out of her feelings, and I'm open to the idea that I could have hurt her unintentionally. Then I try to repair the misunderstanding in record time to alleviate the unease that has penetrated the office environment. In certain subtle respects, this approach is also an easy way out.

While some of my comments start with "I can understand . . . " in an attempt to show empathy for Sallie's current state, my choice of words doesn't address the fact that we reached this impasse because I hadn't understood Sallie's perspective originally. The use of mollifying words forces a semblance of empathy. They don't demonstrate a true grasp and acceptance of Sallie's angry and hurt feelings and of her current need to express them.

In addition, my profuse apologies are so repetitive that they seem automatic. I am too eager to regain Sallie's good graces. By not encouraging Sallie to express a range of emotions in response to the incident, I might give the impression that I can't tolerate and survive her anger.

Apologizing for hurting the patient may be important, but first it's crucial to learn more about the misunderstanding. Example 15.2 illustrates how a more experienced therapist might respond to the empathic lapse.

EXAMPLE 15.2

The more experienced therapist talks with a patient in detail about a recent empathic lapse

SALLIE: Sometimes I feel so independent, and other times I just want to curl up into a little ball and cry.

THERAPIST: So, sometimes you feel like an adult, and other times you feel like a little girl.

SALLIE: (*Looks down at the floor and twists a tissue in her hands.*) I guess so.

THERAPIST: What are you feeling? (*with a gentle look*)

SALLIE: Nothing. I'm just thinking of the work I need to do tonight.

Next Session

SALLIE: I don't have anything to say today.

THERAPIST: (*Nods but does not say anything. I want to allow Sallie's associations to emerge.*)

SALLIE: I am not a little girl! (*Blurts angrily.*)

THERAPIST: Hmm? (*quizzical and concerned look*)

SALLIE: Last session, you said this thing that just wasn't true. Remember when you said that I sometimes act like a little girl?

I don't know. Is that how you see me? I don't even know what to say to you anymore if that's the case.

I can't believe that I have been confiding in you for months, and you don't understand me at all.

THERAPIST: Feeling so misunderstood is upsetting. Can you tell me more? What do you remember of what we both said?

SALLIE: Well, I've just started to feel totally comfortable talking to you. I mean, before last week, I thought I could tell you anything, and then *boom*!

THERAPIST: *Boom?*

SALLIE: Boom, you label me as a little girl! I am coming to therapy to help me grow up and deal with these types of problems. Maybe sometimes I need a little extra help, but I'm not a kid.

THERAPIST: I agree that needing a little extra help doesn't mean that you are a kid. Do you remember any more about the interaction?

SALLIE: Well, all week, I wondered if I should stop therapy. I'd thought you were on my side, and then all of a sudden you start to be so judgmental.

THERAPIST: My comment about feeling like a little girl felt like a judgment?

SALLIE: Of course it did. I am trying so hard to act grown-up and mature in my life. Then you label me with "little girl." It shows me how little you understand me.

THERAPIST: First, I am glad you can tell me this so directly. It sounds like I really did miss the boat, as my mention of "little girl feelings" felt insulting. Even though I did not mean it in an insulting way, my choice of words didn't reflect your efforts to master the problems we have been discussing.

I think it's important to add that I don't see you as a little girl at all. I see how hard you are working to find your path as an adult, and my comment didn't support that growth.

SALLIE: That's true. It really hurt.

THERAPIST: I think you also mentioned wanting to curl into a ball and cry during part of our discussion last week. I wish I had asked you to describe that experience in more detail instead. Perhaps some time you can tell me more about it.

It's to your credit that you let me know how you felt about my comment last week. I hope I won't make such mistakes again, but if I do, I hope you'll tell me right away.

Example 15.2 illustrates procedures that a therapist can employ when reviewing an empathic lapse with a patient. When Sallie starts to relate her disappointment, I don't immediately validate her feelings or move on to another topic as quickly as possible. Instead, I ask her to recall the upsetting events in detail, with the questions: "Can you tell me more? What do you remember of what we both said?"

As I learn about the prior misunderstanding in more detail, I do not share the details of my personal perspective of the preceding event. I focus primarily on Sallie's emotional position to understand why the interaction was so painful for her.

Meanwhile, I try to stay calm and nonjudgmental throughout the experience. After I "get it," I can provide, during the replay, the empathy that was missing the first time around.

AN EMPATHIC LAPSE AS A RESULT OF A THERAPIST'S COUNTERTRANSFERENCE REACTION

Sometimes an empathic lapse occurs when my countertransference—my subjective reaction to the patient—interferes with my ability to respond therapeutically. I find these empathic lapses especially challenging as I need to respond to the patient's needs while simultaneously analyzing my own inner experience.

We've set up an example of a countertransference reaction leading to an empathic lapse in Examples 15.3 and 15.4. When Sallie starts to make some new friends other than Gwen, I'm surprised to find that I am not as pleased as I might have expected. Maybe I feel unconsciously possessive of Sallie after working with her intensively for many months, and I am reluctant to share my special niche as her confidant.

Occasionally I have felt pangs of jealousy when a young adult patient has found a special mentor in her life and has talked repeatedly about how this person is so helpful, unusual, creative, and so forth. Although my patient's comments are evidence of emotional growth, sometimes it's not easy to feel replaced.

I'm sharing this story to encourage you not to disregard these feelings, unappealing as they may be. When these feelings are recognized and processed, the therapy can be protected. They are most troublesome when they are ignored.

When I don't admit my feelings of jealousy to myself in Example 15.3, I unconsciously act on them by criticizing Sallie's new choice of friends.

EXAMPLE 15.3

The therapist's countertransference reaction results in an empathic lapse, and the therapist cannot immediately untangle her own issues from those of the patient

SALLIE: I am so excited! I went to a campus forum sponsored by the local newspaper, and I met some really neat girls. They all live together in a sorority on campus, and they invited me to dinner. I had an amazing time.

There was one girl, Emme, who was especially neat. She was

so nice to me. She's also kinda interested in journalism, but she's actually done something about it. She writes for the campus paper, and, if I get up the guts, I may start working there a little too.

She seems so generous. I needed to get some stuff off campus and she let me borrow her car. Wow! It's hard to believe she might become a new friend. I was so happy all week after meeting her. She's everything I could wish for in a friend. She's incredible!

THERAPIST: Is she incredible on the inside as well? [*I feel a little annoyed at Sallie's news, but I'm not able to recognize my feelings of jealousy. I formulate this question in response to my internal state. If I had been able to process my own feelings independently, I would have chosen a different question that was more protective of Sallie's emotional growth.*]

SALLIE: What do you mean? Emme already seems so different than Gwen. I don't understand. I thought you wanted me to make new friends.

THERAPIST: It just seems it is easy for you to idealize Emme when you hardly know her. [*I am still unaware of any countertransference feelings that are fueling this line of questioning.*]

SALLIE: Dr. Bender, that seems like a weird thing for you to say. Are you prejudiced against sororities?

THERAPIST: Do I sound that way to you?

SALLIE: Yes. I don't know . . . I was so excited about this news. I thought you would be also. Do you think the Greek system is bad?

THERAPIST: Well, let's look at this together. What if I did have a problem with it, and what if I didn't?

SALLIE: I don't know . . . I don't know . . . I just don't know what to say now.

I thought you would be happy for me. Maybe you're right. I don't really know Emme very well yet, even though we've talked every night on the phone this week.

THERAPIST: It's hard for you to hear me state an opinion.

SALLIE: I don't know. I was feeling so happy about this. Now I just feel upset. (*Wipes her eyes.*)

Usually you are happy for me when I am happy. I don't think you have ever acted critical like this before. I don't get it. Did I do something wrong?

THERAPIST: No. It's fine that you have a new friend.

Sallie accurately picks up on my countertransference and is gutsy enough to share her thoughts with me directly. While patients are rarely able to share their thoughts so candidly early in a psychotherapy, we imbued Sallie with this attribute to illustrate this challenging clinical situation.

Unfortunately, while Sallie has the ability to confront me, I'm not up to the challenge. My unconscious worry that Sallie's new friends might replace me fuels my slightly snide, insensitive, and countertherapeutic reactions. The therapy would be better off if I could recognize my true feelings about Sallie's news, and then process them independently of Sallie, either alone or in supervision. A therapist's own therapy is also a haven for understanding countertransference enactments.

Example 15.4 illustrates how a therapist can process a countertransference reaction while simultaneously protecting her patient.

EXAMPLE 15.4

The therapist realizes that her countertransference reaction resulted in some unempathic responses and accepts responsibility for her behavior

SALLIE: I am so excited! . . . (See Example 15.3 for the full text.) . . . It's hard to believe she might become a new friend. I was so happy all week after meeting her. She's everything I could wish for in a friend. She's incredible!

THERAPIST: Is she incredible on the inside as well? [*I feel annoyed and then notice that I feel a little jealous of Sallie's new friends.*]

SALLIE: What do you mean? Emme already seems so different than Gwen. I don't understand. I thought you wanted me to make new friends

THERAPIST: Let me think for a minute. How did you hear what I just said? [*I notice after the words pop out of my mouth that my first comment responded more to my own internal state than to Sallie's comments. I make a mental note to think about this more as I write up my process notes at the end of the session.*]

SALLIE: Well, I am so happy about this new group of friends, and Emme seems especially nice. So far, I don't feel stupid when I'm with Emme, and that happens with Gwen all the time.

Haven't we been working on this idea that I could have better friends for a long time? I don't understand why you said that.

THERAPIST: [*I hear Sallie's point, and I don't want to dismiss her anger.*]

It was a bad choice of words, actually. I agree that we have been working on the idea that you could find more supportive friends. My comment wasn't supportive.

SALLIE: No, it wasn't.

THERAPIST: [*I wait for a moment to allow Sallie to express her frustration.*]

SALLIE: I don't get it. It's not like you to say something sort of mean. Did I do something wrong? Are you mad at me?

THERAPIST: I'm not mad at you, and you certainly didn't do anything wrong. I think my first take on the news was off-base. I did not give you enough credit for your good judgment. It sounds like you have met some nice people who are worth getting to know better.

SALLIE: It is okay for me to talk about my new friends with you, isn't it?

THERAPIST: Absolutely. I'm very interested in hearing about Emme and any other new friend you want to tell me about.

It makes sense, though, that you might feel distrustful after the error I made. If I make another such mistake, I hope you'll let me know about it.

SALLIE: I just don't feel like talking about them anymore today.

THERAPIST: How do you feel about my having made this error and your having to call it to my attention?

SALLIE: Whatever.

THERAPIST: Did I hurt your feelings?

SALLIE: No, it just was a surprise—that's all. I don't expect that type of comment from you.

THERAPIST: I wonder if this has undermined your trust in me. (*sensitively forthright*)

SALLIE: I don't know. Maybe a little. It's just unexpected because we've been talking for weeks about my need for more supportive friends. I thought you would be excited for me.

I don't know. I feel weird talking to you about this.

THERAPIST: What's weird about it for you?

SALLIE: I don't want you to feel bad, but I also didn't like what you said.

THERAPIST: I'm glad you let me know your concerns, but, actually, I welcome your honesty. I think we can both learn a lot if we work this out together.

SALLIE: I don't know. I can't think of anything to say. I'm sorry Dr.

Bender, but I don't want to say something wrong, or have you say something wrong again.

THERAPIST: You didn't say anything wrong. I did. My comment was hurtful. We have been talking about how nice it would be to find some friends other than Gwen. I didn't acknowledge how exciting it feels to be getting to know Emme.

I misunderstood you, but I hope we can work it out. One of the most important lessons in life is to learn how to resolve problems when one person hurts another.

SALLIE: That sounds good, in theory. . . .

THERAPIST: Can you tell me what crossed your mind?

SALLIE: Well, I don't think it is that easy to repair a relationship after a fight. That has been my experience anyway.

THERAPIST: What has been your experience?

SALLIE: Well, when my mom and I fight, for instance . . .

THERAPIST: (*Nods encouragingly.*)

SALLIE: There always seems to be a major rift between us after all our fights. Even the stupid ones.

THERAPIST: Can you give me an example?

SALLIE: Well, a couple weeks ago, I wanted to talk to her about my new friends, and she said she was too busy. I got really angry and hung up. I know I overreacted, but I was really upset at the time.

Anyway, she hasn't called me since. And I don't want to call her, after she dissed me.

THERAPIST: It struck a very sensitive nerve when she wouldn't provide what you needed?

SALLIE: Well, yeah. She never seems too busy to do things for my brother, but if I have a simple request, she has better things to do. Now that we are in a fight, we may not talk to each other for a few weeks. See what I mean? Fights hurt relationships. They don't help them grow.

THERAPIST: Well, I agree with you that the relationship may have trouble growing when the fight stays unresolved. If you would like, maybe we could talk more about your fights with your mother and how they evolve.

SALLIE: I don't know. How can I be sure you won't insult me again?

THERAPIST: You can't right now, but in my experience, a relationship grows in trust if a misunderstanding is processed and resolved.

SALLIE: You think so? I've haven't really experienced that in my relationships.

THERAPIST: I've seen it happen. I hope we can accomplish this together.

SALLIE: How do we start?

THERAPIST: Well, how are you feeling right now?

SALLIE: Kind of overwhelmed. I wish the session were over already.

THERAPIST: The first few times it can feel overwhelming to try to work through a major misunderstanding. Can you tell me more about how you are feeling?

SALLIE: Well, what happens now? I don't really feel like talking about my mother and our stupid fights. I'd rather tell you about this article I agreed to help Emme with. It's for the school paper, but you probably aren't interested.

THERAPIST: Actually, I am very interested.

SALLIE: You are? It's not a big problem. It's more of a success. Is that okay to talk about too?

THERAPIST: Absolutely. I want to hear about anything that you would like to share with me, your successes in addition to your struggles. My first reaction during this session may have made it seem that I wasn't as interested in your achievement—finding Emme as a new friend. I'm sorry for that.

SALLIE: (*excitedly*) Okay. Well, after Emme and I finish this article, I may try to write one on my own. (*Eagerly shares more information about her plans.*)

THERAPIST: (*Nods and smiles.*)

In Example 15.4, I am able to identify my unhelpful countertransference reaction within the session. I can try to understand the details of my reaction after the session is over. Meanwhile, I am able to repair my lapse in understanding with Sallie during our session. While this is the ideal, often the therapy doesn't evolve so smoothly.

Example 15.5 illustrates how I might repair an empathic lapse 1 week after it occurred and effectively respond to Sallie's insistent curiosity about the incident.

EXAMPLE 15.5

After responding unempathically to the patient in a previous sesssion (Example 15.3), the therapist works through her own countertransference reaction and, in the next session, talks with the patient about the interaction

One Week after the Session in Example 15.3

Sallie is talking about her courses for the first 15 minutes of the session. She seems to be avoiding any mention of her new friends.

THERAPIST: I would like to hear more about your new courses, but I wanted to make sure we had a chance to get back to our discussion last week about your new friends.

SALLIE: Oh, it's okay. I have enough other things to talk about. It felt uncomfortable talking about them last week anyway. Let's just forget it.

THERAPIST: Actually I think it is important to discuss. I can appreciate that it was uncomfortable for you last week. As I thought about it later, I realized that I may have missed the boat.

SALLIE: Huh? What do you mean?

THERAPIST: I think you may have felt uncomfortable talking about your friends last week because my reaction wasn't very understanding. If you agree, I'd like to try to talk about it again.

SALLIE: Oh God, do we have to?

THERAPIST: What would it be like to reopen the topic?

SALLIE: I don't know. I just felt like you weren't supportive of my new friends last week, and that was so weird. I thought that was our mutual goal: helping me to find new friends. When I finally make some progress, you didn't trust my choices.

THERAPIST: You were reaching out to new people, and in effect I criticized your growth and courage with a new group of friends. I was wrong to do that.

SALLIE: It means a lot to hear you say that.

THERAPIST: What does it feel like?

SALLIE: Well, you made me so mad last week. I almost skipped this week's session.

I knew you didn't understand, and then I wondered if you disapproved of me. You just couldn't see my point of view. Like I said, I almost cancelled our meeting today. I didn't really want to come back.

THERAPIST: It took self-discipline and courage for you to come to your session today. It was understandably hard to return after I disappointed you.

I'm glad you made it. By coming, we have the chance to work this out together.

SALLIE: Usually, you let me talk about what is important to me, but you were so different last week. I don't know what to talk about now.

THERAPIST: You are right. My intention is to talk with you about whatever feels important to you, and last week I didn't do that. When you brought up Emme for the first time, my response wasn't very sensitive or useful.

SALLIE: Yeah, you made things worse instead of better. That's never happened before. Did I do something wrong? Why did you do that?

THERAPIST: [*Being fully open wouldn't respond to Sallie's needs.*] You did nothing wrong at all. My comments were off-base, and they did make things worse intead of better. That is why I wanted to make sure we talked about it today.

SALLIE: Yeah, you don't usually make comments like this. It would just help me to know why it happened.

THERAPIST: How would it help you?

SALLIE: I don't know. I feel a little worried.

THERAPIST: Worried about what?

SALLIE: Well, are you okay? Did my problems upset you?

THERAPIST: Did I seem upset last week?

SALLIE: I don't know. Maybe a little bit.

THERAPIST: Perhaps I may have seemed upset to you last week, because my comments weren't supportive. But it's important for you to know that I said the things I said because my focus was off. [*Sharing the details of my reaction wouldn't be therapeutic. It had more to do with me than with Sallie.*]

Now I'm encouraged that you were able to tell me your feelings so directly. You're right. I wasn't being very helpful last week.

SALLIE: Well, I don't want our relationship to change because I've told you that you did something wrong.

THERAPIST: The misunderstanding makes our relationship feel more tenuous?

SALLIE: Yeah, sort of.

THERAPIST: I think we'll learn more over time about this concern, but I view our relationship as stronger for weathering a troubling interaction. If I ever misunderstand anything in the future, I hope you will tell me as you did this time.

SALLIE: (*beaming*) Sure, you know it seems pretty brave to me that you brought last week's spat back up. I'm glad we talked about it.

THERAPIST: And you were brave too.

SALLIE: Yeah, I guess so. Maybe you are right.

Many individuals seek therapy because they have experienced a lack of empathy from important figures in their life. One of the healing aspects of psychotherapy is the experience of feeling safe, affirmed, and understood. This experience is fortified when a misunderstanding is worked through rather than denied or deflected. Once Sallie has experienced working through a misunderstanding with me, she might feel more capable of talking openly and honestly after a disagreement with other significant people in her life.

UNCOVERING A POTENTIAL EMPATHIC LAPSE

While Example 15.5 illustrates a potentially stressful situation, it is easy in one respect: Sallie doesn't deny that I made a hurtful comment. Rather than being shy or indirect, she tells me exactly which of my statements bothered her and why. Many patients aren't this direct.

Sometimes, I wonder whether I committed an empathic lapse during a session and missed the patient's cues that my comments were hurtful. In my early days in psychiatry I would often worry that I had caused irreparable emotional damage when I critiqued my work after the session was over. Even if my patient hadn't seemed particularly bent out of shape during the hour, I would start to worry about my responses until I reached supervision to confess my most recent "mistakes." Words that had felt direct and sincere at the time seemed judgmental and harsh when I reviewed my notes. Questions that had appeared crucially insightful sounded like unnecessary, insensitive interruptions. Now and again, a supervisor would also specifically criticize a statement I had made, fueling my anxiety that I had hurt my patient emotionally.

Lucky for me, most of my supervisors were extremely supportive when I started sharing my concerns. Here are some of their tips: First, if a therapist makes a less than ideal comment during a session and the patient *doesn't* react, it is impossible to assess how the patient experienced the moment. (This is a situation different from Example 15.3, in which I misunderstand Sallie during the session, and she immediately expresses disappointment.) Second, if the patient didn't seem taken aback by my comment when I made it, it is not therapeutic for me to confess to a possible empathic lapse at our next meeting. Since I don't possess psychic powers, I have no idea how last week's statement was interpreted by the patient. My patient may not even remember the comment I wish I had never uttered.

If I'm really concerned, I might ask a patient at a natural pause in the session how she experienced a certain part of last week's meeting. If she brushes it off, I follow suit. In my experience, the statements that I wish I had never uttered are rarely the ones that my patients tag as empathic lapses.

Another tactic is to listen carefully during the next session to see if Sallie alludes to a potential empathic lapse from the previous meeting. If Sallie shares her reaction directly, I am home free and can use the advice outlined in the previous examples.

Let's pretend that Sallie had not expressed her frustration when I wasn't very supportive about her new friendship with Emme. As I review my notes in supervision, I start to wonder whether my comments could have been upsetting to her. Example 15.6 illustrates how to handle the situation in the following session if Sallie drops some subtle hints about a prior empathic lapse.

EXAMPLE 15.6

The patient alludes to an empathic lapse in the previous session, and the therapist helps her talk about it directly

SALLIE: So, I had a horrible week.

THERAPIST: Oh (*concerned look*), what happened?

SALLIE: I don't know really. I just felt lonely all week. I didn't see any of those new friends I told you about. Maybe I avoided them a little bit.

THERAPIST: How did you avoid them?

SALLIE: Well, I didn't hang out where I thought I might see them. I just felt so exhausted. You know, normal college burnout.

THERAPIST: Do you have an understanding of what might be burning you out?

SALLIE: Not really. I just feel very out of it this week.

THERAPIST: Did anything happen in our last session that made your week more difficult?

SALLIE: Not really. . . . I don't know.

THERAPIST: (*Quiet, encouraging look*)

SALLIE: Well, I did wonder about one comment that you made.

THERAPIST: Could you tell me about it?

SALLIE: Well, remember I told you that I had met this really nice girl, Emme, and I was really excited to have a new friend?

THERAPIST: (*Nods.*)

SALLIE: Well, you said a weird thing.

THERAPIST: What was the weird thing?

SALLIE: Well, you said something about how Emme might be superficial. I don't really remember the words.

THERAPIST: Do you remember my comment specifically?

SALLIE: Yes, it was something that Emme might just look good on the outside. I got this feeling that you didn't want me to be friends with her.

THERAPIST: As I think back on it now, I can see how my comment might have felt upsetting. How did it affect you?

SALLIE: Well, I respect your opinion. You're probably right that Emme isn't that great. I was just really excited after I met her.

THERAPIST: While I appreciate that you respect my opinion, I think my comment was misguided. If you were really excited after meeting Emme, she is someone worth getting to know better.

SALLIE: You really think so?

THERAPIST: I do, and I'm sorry that I wasn't able to express this message first and foremost.

SALLIE: I am too, but it means a lot that you told me this.

During the first part of the session in Example 15.6, Sallie alludes to her disappointment in vague, derivative terms. My open-ended question acknowledges that the therapy could have contributed to her distress, and Sallie slowly starts to talk about her discontent.

What should I do if Sallie does not attribute any of her current distress to the previous therapy session? I could repeat a couple of comments such as "I wonder if anything in the therapy could have contributed to your stressful week?" but if Sallie doesn't respond, I would not pursue the topic. Forcing an issue is not therapeutic. First, I can't be certain that Sallie's distress is a result of an interaction that occurred in the therapy. While the therapy hour is a significant part of a patient's life, it is only 1 hour in a busy week. I need to avoid overemphasizing its importance. Second, Sallie may not be ready to talk about the misunderstanding so directly. If this is the case, it is enough that I express my interest in talking about our interaction. I can hope that sometime in the future she may be ready to express her feelings more openly. In the meantime, we can focus on the issues that Sallie feels comfortable talking about in more detail.

Empathic lapses are challenging, especially for the beginning therapist. As we have indicated, an honest approach of reviewing the incident, responding to the replay empathically, and taking responsibility as indicated may ultimately result in a therapeutic experience for the patient. Again, the goal is not to pretend to be the perfect and invariably sensitive therapist. The best therapists try to help the patient work through misunderstandings as part of the emotional growth process.

The therapist can also evolve and mature through these often distressing experiences. She can learn to keep cool in the face of hostility instead of acting in an offensive or defensive manner. She can learn to accept that empathic lapses occur and that they needn't be the end of a psychotherapy. Finally, situations in which we are insufficiently empathic can serve as indicators, pointing us toward facets of our own inner life that need attention.

Through our own efforts at introspection or with the help of colleagues, supervisors, or our own therapists, we can develop strength where there had been vulnerability. Over time, the recognition of our areas of limitation can help us develop greater maturity, serenity, and skill.

Key words: countertransference, empathic failure, empathy, impasses, intersubjectivity, misunderstanding, psychotherapy, rapport, therapeutic alliance, trust

16

Transference and Countertransference

As human beings, we learn from our experiences with others. We transfer expectations based on important relationships to new individuals that we meet. This phenomenon is called transference. One feature of emotional health is the capacity to revise expectations of relationships appropriately as we expand our experiences with people.

Sometimes unconscious transference can impair psychological functioning. When transference enters the psychotherapeutic relationship and is discussed openly by therapist and patient, profound learning and maturation may result.

Therapists can also transfer their own expectations to their patients. They also react to their patients emotionally (countertransference). Courageous recognition of those feelings combined with constructive examination can diminish obstacles to the patient's therapeutic progress. In many instances, such introspection may reinvigorate the psychological treatment.

Transference is a form of social memory. Experiences with primary people from our childhood, usually our parents, teach us how to relate to others outside the immediate family. Either consciously or unconsciously, we transfer expectations that we carry from past interactions onto new relationships. This transference effect may be subtle or dramatic. For example: A patient with a supportive family may expect authority figures to be helpful and comforting. A patient who has experienced neglect and abuse on the homefront may assume that this experience will continue in other venues, personal and professional.

When a therapist divulges very little information about herself and doesn't make any personal demands, the transference from patient to therapist is more easily observed than with many other relationships. With an empathic approach, the therapist can use the transference to increase the patient's understanding of herself.

Naturally, therapists also respond emotionally to their patients. This phenomenon is called countertransference. Countertransference reactions can be intense and may feel distracting to a novice therapist who is trying to pay attention to her patient's concerns. If understood, these reactions may inform the treatment rather than pollute it, providing emotional data that would be otherwise unobtainable.

TRANSFERENCE IN THE FIRST MEETING

While a patient's transference toward her therapist tends to deepen as the therapy progresses, it may begin with their first contact. For instance, during a first session, a patient may have a strong emotional reaction—favorable or unfavorable—to a personal feature of the therapist, such as gender, age, or skin color. Since the patient has just barely met the therapist, her opinion is probably a transference reaction, because it is based on past experiences. If the reaction is favorable—for example, the patient wanted to see a young female therapist and the therapist is young, female, and reminds the patient of her comforting sister—it is unlikely that the issue will ever need to be discussed. On the other hand, if the patient has a strong aversive first impression of the therapist, the treatment will benefit if this issue is addressed as soon as it becomes evident.

Example 16.1 illustrates how a therapist can attempt to forge a therapeutic alliance with a new patient who has an aversive transference reaction during the first session.

EXAMPLE 16.1

The therapist responds appropriately to a patient with a strongly aversive first impression

First Meeting

THERAPIST: Hello, I am Dr. Bender.

SALLIE: My goodness, you are so young!

THERAPIST: What?

SALLIE: I expected someone older. You don't look older than 25. I'm sorry. I was just hoping for someone with some more experience.

THERAPIST: More experience?

SALLIE: Well, you sounded older over the phone. I just wanted to see a therapist with more life experience than I have. You know, with wisdom—no offense, I hope.

THERAPIST: No offense taken. I can imagine it is quite a disappointment meeting me if you were hoping for someone older. [*Although I want to tell Sallie that I am older than I look, I resist the urge.*]

SALLIE: Yes, it is. Could I switch to someone else in the clinic?

THERAPIST: It might be possible to arrange that. If I know a bit more about what you are looking for and what brought you to therapy in the first place, I can make a more informed referral.

How would you feel about meeting with me for a session or two to talk about these issues? Then, I can use this information to find you a clinician you may feel more comfortable with.

SALLIE: Okay, but I'm pretty sure I'll want to switch after the first few meetings.

THERAPIST: I can understand your concern. It is important to try to find a therapist you feel comfortable with, so he or she can be helpful to you.

In Example 16.1, I don't take Sallie's comments personally. Her preference for older clinicians predates her meeting with me and may be in response to previous interactions with younger and older helping figures in her life. The offer of the extended consultation followed by a referral to an older clinician is empathic and clinically strategic. The plan validates Sallie's wish for an older provider, while the future meetings give us the opportunity to work together briefly. While some unfavorable initial transference reactions are formidable, a large percentage dissipate once the patient feels validated, respected, and understood. It is possible that once we get started, our therapeutic alliance will evolve and the referral to another clinician will be unnecessary.

TRANSFERENCE IN AN ONGOING TREATMENT

Usually, transferential issues, when the patient expects that the therapist will act like a previously encountered important person in her life, emerge as the treatment evolves. Great therapeutic gains can be made if these matters can be discussed openly and sensitively. The therapist can also use her own feelings toward the patient, the countertransference, to inform this discussion further.

The interaction requires some clinical finesse. First timers may be subject to some of the common difficulties outlined in Example 16.2.

EXAMPLE 16.2

The therapist experiences a transference reaction as a personal attack and responds countertherapeutically

SALLIE: I've been thinking about the possibility of changing majors, but like I've said before, I'm too scared to disappoint my mother. I don't know what to do.

THERAPIST: Can you say more about what you are scared of?

SALLIE: Well, I want my mother to be proud of me. That isn't abnormal, right? I'm her daughter who might get rich after graduation. I'm her future CEO. You should see her beam when she talks about this.
    I don't want to mess with it. It means so much to me that she cares.

THERAPIST: (*Nods.*)

SALLIE: I don't want to talk to her about the fact that I might be sort of interested in becoming a journalist.

THERAPIST: Hmm-mm. (*Nods in understanding.*)

SALLIE: Dr. Bender, I just don't feel comfortable talking to her about this, no matter what you say.

THERAPIST: [*I hadn't felt a need to force Sallie to confront her mother, and I feel miffed that she would assume that I would be so directive.*] You can do what you want. It's your life. I don't feel the need to direct your life.

SALLIE: Umm, I know. I just thought you might want me to be more direct with her about my feelings.

THERAPIST: Well, you don't have to worry about that with me. I am more interested in helping you find the direction that feels best to you.

Next Session

SALLIE: I felt really terrible this week. I didn't sleep well at all last night. I kept the lights on at night. I think I told you that I do this sometimes when I'm feeling stressed.
    Don't ask me why I'm feeling down. I have no idea, and I know that is your next question.

THERAPIST: This one is hard to figure out?

SALLIE: Yeah. I don't get it. Don't get mad at me though. That would make it feel worse.

THERAPIST: Do you feel that I'm mad at you?

SALLIE: Well, you don't seem mad now, but I thought you might have been a little aggravated at me last week.

THERAPIST: Aggravated? Why would I be aggravated? [*I did feel a little aggravated last week, but I have no idea how to address this with Sallie.*]

SALLIE: Well, I know you said that you didn't care if I talked with my mother about my career worries, but I guess I don't really believe you. I know that it would be in my best interest to talk to her. I feel sort of stupid that I just complain to you about my problems with her but never talk to her about it directly.

THERAPIST: Can you say more?

SALLIE: Well, I kind of worry that I might be disappointing you because I'm too scared to talk to her. Meanwhile, you must be bored of hearing me come in here and obsess about the fact that I don't like my major.

THERAPIST: [*I remember now that I was annoyed last week when Sallie made a similar statement. I still don't understand why she thinks I would be as directive as her mother when I have tried so hard to help her find her own way. I start to worry about my ability as a therapist.*] Yes, I know you feel that, but I don't understand why. I am more interested in helping you find your own direction, not choosing it for you. (*frustrated tone*)

SALLIE: I'm sorry. I know you said that last week also. I just still feel a little worried about it.

THERAPIST: [*I suddenly understand Sallie's reaction in terms of transference. To assuage my increasing feeling of insecurity about my therapeutic prowess, I present my next comment with great authority.*] Why of course! You feel like I have expectations of you just like your mother does!

SALLIE: What do you mean?

THERAPIST: Well, you feel that your mother wouldn't care for you unless you follow her agenda. Now you feel that about me too! It all makes perfect sense. [*I feel less helpless after I've made my interpretation. I don't have an understanding of my own countertransference, and how it is fueling my current insensitive approach.*]

SALLIE: Umm, well, maybe a little bit.

THERAPIST: I think we have figured this out. So can you tell me what it would be like to talk to your mother about changing your major?

SALLIE: I just don't want to. I hope that's okay. (*Seems timid.*) I don't really get what you are saying anyway. I know that you aren't my mother.

THERAPIST: Yes, of course, but since you've experienced your mother as making demands on you, you've started to feel that way with me as well. [*I feel proud of my theory and don't notice Sallie's increasing discomfort.*]

SALLIE: No, not really. (*Averts her eyes.*)

THERAPIST: Well, just think about how much sense it makes. It's very hard for you to assert yourself with confident women, but that's okay. We'll work on that.

SALLIE: (*Seems embarrassed.*) Umm, whatever you say. I guess you know best. You are the doctor.

THERAPIST: This sounds familiar to me. With women in authority positions, you always assume they know best rather than listening to yourself. It is your way of trying to maintain a connection, but it means you always have to be in the subservient role. [*I still don't notice Sallie's increasing withdrawal.*]

SALLIE: (*Tears arise, and she doesn't say anything.*)

Sallie's expectations that I will act in a directive manner like her mother are an example of transference. When I don't recognize this phenomenon early in Example 16.2, my understanding of Sallie's insecurities is limited: ["I hadn't felt a need to force Sallie to confront her mother, and I feel miffed that she would assume that I would be so directive."].

As the example continues, I identify Sallie's expectation (or transference) that she needs to follow the guidance of woman in authority to maintain the relationship's emotional connection. My confrontational manner is an attempt to assuage my own feelings of inexpertise. Even if my interpretation may be factually correct, my method of presentation combined with bad timing is more of an emotional assault. Sallie doesn't gain emotional understanding from the interaction. Instead, she withdraws during my subsequent line of questioning.

My comments in Example 16.2 also illustrate two important psychological phenomena: countertransference enactment and complementary identification. Sallie becomes a target of a countertransference enactment when my unresolved insecurities are expressed outwardly in a way that affects her. The complementary identification occurs when I inadvertently mimic Sallie's mother's authoritative female role after all.

Example 16.3 illustrates a more therapeutic intervention in response to Sallie's concerns.

EXAMPLE 16.3

The patient's transference reaction is used to inform and to advance the therapy

SALLIE: I've been thinking about the possibility of changing majors, but like I've said before, I'm too scared to disappoint my mother. It's such a difficult situation.

THERAPIST: Can you say more about what you are scared of?

SALLIE: Well, I want my mother to be proud of me. That isn't abnormal, right? I don't want to mess anything up. It means so much to me that she cares.

THERAPIST: (*Nods.*)

SALLIE: I don't want to talk to her about the fact that I might be more interested in journalism.

THERAPIST: Can you say any more?

SALLIE: I just don't think you understand that talking to her is too risky.

THERAPIST: Do you feel that I want you to talk with her?

SALLIE: Maybe. You've pointed out that I've never talked to her about my worries, and I figured you wouldn't have said that unless you thought it was a good idea. I know you want what's best for me, but I'm just not up to it.

THERAPIST: [*I feel annoyed that Sallie would think I would act in such a directive way, but then decide to understand this response as an informative piece of countertransference. It is interesting that Sallie would assume that I would be directive, as her mother is. Her assumptions are incorrect because I hadn't been thinking that Sallie should confront her mother. Could Sallie be misunderstanding her mother as well? Food for thought.*] How long have you felt that I wanted you to talk with your mother?

SALLIE: I don't know. Maybe the last couple of weeks or so, since I've been telling you more about my mom. I just assumed that you would want me to confront her if it bothered me so much. It must be annoying to hear me complain without actively trying to change the situation. I've just been a little worried about it.

THERAPIST: [*With supervision, I had felt comfortable continuing to explore Sallie's concerns rather than pushing her to act. Sallie's assumptions about my reactions continue to be inaccurate. I suppress a desire to correct her impression that I have a covert agenda. There is more information to be gained if I continue to learn more about Sallie's perspective.*] Can you tell me more about your worries?

SALLIE: Well, I'm worried about what you'll think if I don't do what you want, even if it is the best thing for me. I respect you so much, and I don't want to disappoint you.

Last week you asked me something about following my dream. I don't know. It made me feel weird. But, I don't want you to feel bad about it. I know you just want the best for me. I just felt sort of pushed after you said that. That's my fault though. I'm the spineless jellyfish here.

THERAPIST: You are letting me off the hook here. It might feel easier to blame yourself rather than to stick with your gut reaction: that the comments I made last week felt directive and weren't helpful. [*I'm trying to respond in a way that validates Sallie's experience without overtly expressing an opinion about my wishes for her future.*]

SALLIE: Yes. I'm worried you might get upset if I don't follow your advice and do things your way.

THERAPIST: If we had different approaches to an issue, would that feel worrisome to you?

SALLIE: Well, sure. I like you and I want you to like me.

THERAPIST: Do you feel that I might not like you if our opinions differed?

SALLIE: Umm, well maybe. You might get mad at me if I didn't follow your advice.

THERAPIST: Mad at you?

SALLIE: Maybe. Well, I don't know. Like I said, I'm mainly worried that you would be upset at me if I don't meet your expectations.

THERAPIST: Are you worried that I would be upset at you if you follow your own beliefs?

SALLIE: Yeah, but it's not a new feeling for me. It's my life with Gwen. I always do what she wants me to do. Otherwise, she's not as interested in spending time with me.

THERAPIST: Do you experience this feeling with anyone else?

SALLIE: No. Not really with anyone that I can think of.

THERAPIST: Do you ever feel this way with anyone in your immediate family?

SALLIE: Umm, well maybe with my mother.

THERAPIST: How so?

SALLIE: Well, you know that I worry about disagreeing with my mother about my future career because I don't want her to be disappointed in me.

THERAPIST: To maintain the closeness, you bury your own wishes?

SALLIE: Yes, but that's just the way it is. I need to learn to deal with it.

THERAPIST: I understand that it is quite a dilemma. Tell me if I am understanding it correctly. You try to ignore your own wishes with your mother because the relationship feels less secure when there is a disagreement. Does that fit to you?

SALLIE: Yes, but it's not that simple.

THERAPIST: Tell me more. What part doesn't feel right to you?

SALLIE: Well, I do worry that my mom might get angry if I disagree with her. But that's not the whole story. I also love the attention I get from her when we do agree about important things. I'm not just avoiding something that feels scary. I also don't want to mess with something that feels so right.

THERAPIST: That makes sense. Thank you for clarifying this for me. Your mother's attention is understandably so valuable to you.

SALLIE: (Nods.)

THERAPIST: Perhaps mine is too.

SALLIE: You mean that your attention is valuable to me?

THERAPIST: (Nods.)

SALLIE: Umm, I guess so, otherwise I wouldn't be so worried about us having different opinions.

THERAPIST: I think it's important that you know that I'm not a bit mad at you for anything. I think it's fine that you've chosen not to talk to your mother about your interest in journalism at this time. Our goal is to enable you to figure out what feels right for you.

SALLIE: It helps to hear that.

THERAPIST: I'm glad, but even if it helps to hear that, your fears of disagreeing with me may not disappear right away. I hope we can keep discussing any worries you might have. We'll see what we can learn together by talking about it openly.

Example 16.3 illustrates how an explanation of transference can flow naturally from a discussion of the patient's concerns. First, Sallie and I talk extensively about her fear that I am disappointed in her. Gradually, we understand how her worries about my reaction are derived from her prior experiences with her mother.

Ultimately, the resolution of our personal conflict will probably have a highly therapeutic impact. By modeling empathic and open communication, I want Sallie to experience firsthand how to work through difficulties within a relationship.

A single conversation won't put Sallie's worries to rest. To work through this issue, we will need to talk about it repeatedly in slightly varied contexts from different emotional angles. It will probably take time before there is any substantial emotional change.

WHEN TALK OF TRANSFERENCE IS DESTABILIZING

In general, a psychotherapy evolves as the therapist and patient focus together on the patient's transference reaction. With some patients though, namely those with impaired reality testing, talking openly about the transference may precipitate a decrease in functioning rather than an increase in insight. As illustrated in Example 16.4 with Candice Jones, I change therapeutic tactics if a patient's reality testing becomes impaired during a transference discussion.

EXAMPLE 16.4

The therapist moves the focus away from the transference when the patient becomes paranoid

In previous sessions, Candice described her father as manipulative and devaluing.

I have taken down a framed poster in the office after it cracked, without providing any replacement art.

CANDICE: Oh, you decided to remove the picture of the water lilies by the doorway. . . .

THERAPIST: Yes.

CANDICE: The walls seem so naked to me now. I do understand the purpose of the change, though. It's not lost on me.

THERAPIST: What?

CANDICE: Well, I know we don't have an egalitarian relationship. You are the one with the power, because I am coming to you for help. Without the art, it is even more obvious that I am the patient. It's a rather antiseptic move, Dr. Bender. Even if you are trying to be more professional, it felt much safer when you actually decorated your office.

THERAPIST: [*Candice's comments are increasingly disorganized and paranoid, but I think it can't hurt to validate her experience.*] So it feels less safe and less equal without the poster?

CANDICE: Oh, it's not that big a deal. I know this is part of your work in order to help focus all the attention on me and all my failings. I can handle it. But you should know this for your other patients. They may not be able to tell you their feelings so openly. But I know this is all part of your treatment plan.

THERAPIST: My treatment plan?

CANDICE: Well, empty walls help patients have trauma flashbacks. The new decor will help you get material.

THERAPIST: [*Candice is clearly decompensating as she transfers expectations from some other relationship onto my change in office decoration. Her associations are less reality-based and more paranoid with each open-ended question. I move to a more reality-based and cognitive approach.*] Actually, I don't have those intentions. The poster's frame cracked, and I am trying either to replace it or to find another poster to take its place.

CANDICE: You don't have an ulterior motive with your new sparse decorating scheme?

THERAPIST: No. No ulterior motive at all. But your point is well taken that the office looks a little bare without the poster to brighten it up. [*I support the part of Candice's opinion that is more reality-based.*]

CANDICE: Yes, I really did like that picture. [*The paranoid associations cease.*]

Transference explorations are relatively unstructured and can be emotionally evocative. For patients with a poor grasp on reality, this approach can be disinhibiting and destabilizing. For patients like Candice Jones, a more cognitive approach is appropriate to maintain the therapeutic connection and to maximize emotional functioning.

COUNTERTRANSFERENCE AND AUTOGNOSIS

Countertransference reactions range as widely as their transference counterparts. Some of them are challenging. Feeling angry, saddened, or helpless in response to a patient's dilemma may be difficult to tolerate and to process. A novice clinician may be inclined to suppress the reaction. While this is an understandable emotional response, the unanalyzed feelings may subtly alter the therapist's perspective of the patient's concerns. In turn, the therapy may be affected detrimentally. On the other hand, if the countertransference feelings are understood, the therapy may benefit. "Autognosis" refers to this kind of self-knowledge.

The therapist's favorable transference to the patient may also affect the treatment. For example, I might look forward to working with one patient in particular because she reminds me of my best friend from elementary school. This response of mine might lead me to underestimate the patient's vulnerabilities and difficulties.

Often, countertransference reactions are subtle. Sometimes within a session I become aware of an unexpected feeling that comes on quickly and powerfully. The patient may be unconsciously manipulating the situation to induce me to share her emotional experience, an occurrence known as concurrent identification. If I can recognize this, I can use this information to shape my intervention.

EXAMPLE 16.5

The therapist notes her own increasing feeling of helplessness in the session and uses the experience to shape her next intervention

SALLIE: Dr. Bender, I really don't think this therapy is helping at all. I understand my dilemma now. Like you said, it feels overwhelming to assert myself with my mother when I am afraid of losing her approval. But so what? I don't feel any better. I'm no expert, of course, but I don't see where this therapy is going.

THERAPIST: [*All of a sudden, I feel at a loss for words.*] Umm, well, how long have you been feeling this?

SALLIE: Oh, I feel it every now and then. Sometimes I feel like I am getting better, and then other times I just don't see the point. So I sit here and talk about my problems. Whoop-de-do. I can talk about my problems forever. That doesn't mean that my problems are going to change.

THERAPIST: [*I feel helpless as Sallie talks about her experience. I wonder if we may be experiencing the same emotional state. I use this information to guide my next line of questioning.*] With all the work you have been doing, do you feel rather helpless with the slow improvement?

SALLIE: Yes, I guess I do.

THERAPIST: Do you have any understanding of why the helplessness is so prevalent right now?

SALLIE: Well, it's nearing the end of the school year, and next year I'll be a senior. I guess the issue we are talking about is really coming to a head. After I graduate, I plan to go to business school, and the whole idea makes me feel nauseous.

THERAPIST: It's so difficult to feel stuck between your mother's wants and your own.

SALLIE: It is. I don't know what to do about it. I know I need to make a change in order to feel better, but I haven't figured out what that will be yet.

THERAPIST: The conflict has been with you for a long time, so it's not surprising that we'll need more time to find a resolution. [*offering reasonable hope*]

A concurrent identification occurs in Example 16.5 when my feelings of helplessness mirror Sallie's emotional state. I use my experience to guide my approach with Sallie. After validating her feelings, the content of the session deepens. As it turns out, Sallie's true concerns center on her dilemma involving her mother more than the efficacy of the treatment.

For a therapist, it's not always as clear-cut and easy to tolerate one's internal emotional state as it appeared in Example 16.5. For example, anger at a patient may not evaporate after a private acknowledgment that it exists.

In such a circumstance I try to express my emotions internally without hurting the patient. Directed fantasy is one way to dispel difficult emotions during or after a difficult interaction with a patient. For instance, if I feel very angry at a devaluing and narcissistic patient, I might imagine yelling or fighting with the patient to express my frustration. By expressing my feelings in fantasy, it may be easier to act professionally and appropriately during trying clinical moments.

It takes knowledge and experience to process one's emotions while simultaneously attending to the patient. I may postpone the fantasy for a private moment to make sure none of the content from my internal imagery trickles inadvertently into the treatment. The use of fantasies is strategic; using my imagination makes it less likely that I will act out my suppressed anger.

Now and then, a therapist's internal reactions to a patient are too intense to be contained simply with a directed fantasy. In these situations, a therapist can access supervision and her own therapy if her reactions toward a patient are infecting a treatment rather than informing it. Supervision is nearly always provided by training programs. Relationships with supervisors can sometimes be continued after graduation. If one moves to another city after training has been completed, competent supervisors can be recommended by professional organizations or by local training institutions. Therapists for the therapist can also be recommmended by these sources.

In order to process the complicated emotional reactions that are a regular part of being a psychotherapist, the clinician needs to take special care of herself. By supporting one's self emotionally, an individual's ability to focus on others will increase. Emotional resilience increases if one takes time to think through difficult situations independently or with supervision. Taking meaningful time in mutual relationships with friends, partners, or relatives, and spending time in activities that bring satisfaction and joy are necessary to maintain psychological health. Knowing one's self well and maintaining one's inner health must be given high priorities in order to preserve one's ability to listen to others carefully, empathically, and effectively.

Key words: autognosis, complementary identification, concurrent identification, countertransference, countertransference enactment, defensiveness, directed fantasies, directed imagery, ego boundaries, empathy, enactment, expectations, fantasies, here and now, idealization, illusions, interpretation, intersubjectivity, patterns of relationship, premature interpretations, psychotherapy, reality testing, tranference, unresolved problems

17

Termination

Termination is the ending phase of therapy. A mature termination is one in which the goals of therapy have been attained. Premature terminations occur when therapy must end for other reasons. Like other separations in life, the ending of therapy may evoke strong feelings, both in the clinician and in the patient. Skillful conduct of this part of therapy can have an emotionally strengthening effect on the therapist as well as on the patient.

It wasn't easy saying good-bye to all of my patients during the last 4 weeks of my training in adult psychiatry. Even though the therapeutic relationships were professional, the separations evoked myriad feelings.

Two parallel processes emerged. I would talk at length with my patients about their experience of the treatment's ending and then rush off to supervision to express how I was coping with it. The extra emotional support was necessary. Until I had independently processed my own perspective, I couldn't fully concentrate on my patient's concerns. Similarly, in this chapter, we pay equal attention to both the patient's and the therapist's needs as we review the process of termination.

WHEN DOES TERMINATION OCCUR?

Patients who drop out of therapy without warning are quitting treatment, not terminating care. (For an approach to a patient who leaves treatment abruptly, see Chapter 10.) When a therapy has had time to develop, its ending, known as a termination, takes on a whole new meaning. In the best circumstances, a mature termination begins when a patient and I realize that she has resolved the main difficulties that brought her to therapy. The parting doesn't feel forced, because the patient is ready to apply independently the emotional knowledge and competence that she has acquired. Although each person's rate of progress in therapy is unique, it takes time—often years—to accomplish the clinical gains necessary for a mature termination.

Since training blocks for psychotherapists usually run for 2 or 3 years, many clinicians won't complete a long-term dynamic psychotherapy as a trainee. Geographical moves or graduations (by the trainee or by the patient) actually make premature terminations the norm early in one's career. Patients deserve to hear this information. We recommend that trainees inform their patients when they will be leaving the clinic at a treatment's onset, as we have illustrated in Example 3.5.

Our first examples consider how to discuss a premature treatment termination with the patient if it is initiated by the clinician's circumstances. The subsequent examples illustrate how the treatment might end if a geographical move by the patient necessitates an early ending to the therapy. Much of the information presented can be applied to mature terminations as well.

THE THERAPIST'S LEAVING LEADS TO A PREMATURE TERMINATION

While I was tempted to keep "forgetting" to tell my patients that I would be leaving the clinic in a few months at the end of my residency, the delay would have been a therapeutic error. Many patients appreciate the time to prepare for a good-bye. It often feels even more painful to be faced with an unexpected separation with no time to process the event.

If the therapy must end prematurely because I need to leave the patient, I share the news approximately 6 months ahead of time. Knowing the exit date may allow the patient to identify and to solidify gains made in the therapy. We'll have ample time to discuss the range of feelings that emerge as the ending approaches.

It's easy to feel guilty about leaving a patient. Example 17.1 illustrates the subtle and not-so-subtle ways in which the ambivalent therapist may overcompensate during the remaining treatment time.

EXAMPLE 17.1

The therapist is unable to maintain a focus on the patient and steps out of her professional role after announcing that she will be leaving the city in 6 months

15 Minutes into the Session

THERAPIST: I have some news I need to tell you today.

SALLIE: Oh, what?

THERAPIST: Well, in July I will be leaving Boston.

SALLIE: Oh, okay. (*nonchalance*) So when is your last week here exactly?

THERAPIST: I will be leaving the last week in June.

SALLIE: Where are you going?

THERAPIST: I will be moving to Florida. I know it's unexpected news. I hope you can feel free to share any reactions you may have in the upcoming months.

SALLIE: Oh, I don't need months to tell you how I feel. I don't care that much. People move on; I understand that. I can see someone else at the clinic, can't I?

THERAPIST: Yes, I can set you up with a referral to continue therapy after I leave. But what about us?

SALLIE: What do you mean?

THERAPIST: Well, we've worked together for almost 3 years now. What will it be like to stop?

SALLIE: I already told you. I wish you well, but I won't crumble or anything without you.

Something interesting did happen at school today though. . . . (*Voice trails off.*)

THERAPIST: Moving away from the fact we will be stopping?

SALLIE: What?

THERAPIST: I just think it might be easier to talk about school than the fact that our relationship will be ending.

SALLIE: No. Six months is far, far away. I probably will be ready to stop then anyway.

THERAPIST: Is it so easy for you to give up on our relationship?

SALLIE: Whatever. . . .

THERAPIST: [*I feel guilty about leaving Sallie, and then uncomfortable with Sallie's indifference. I decide to share my own personal feelings about the termination as it might help Sallie open up.*] I do feel very bad about leaving the area, as we can't continue to work together. I know it is disruptive for me to leave you just as you are making progress with the issues that have been concerning you. I will really miss working with you.

SALLIE: Oh, you don't need to say that. You are paid to work with me. I knew that you would leave sooner or later anyway. You told me that you were in training during one of our first meetings.

In Example 17.1, Sallie reacts to our unexpected upcoming termination date with a veil of denial and indifference. Her response may be both emotionally protective and retaliatory.

I don't recognize that her reaction may be a defense against possibly intolerable feelings of abandonment and loss. Instead, I repeatedly move the topic back to my upcoming exit. I try to induce Sallie to express a set of emotions that is more in tune with my own feelings. The fortitude of Sallie's defenses, basically the "I-don't-care" stance, is strengthened.

Then, because Sallie's indifference is so unexpected, and because I feel so guilty for ending the therapy prematurely, I interject my own personal emotions about the upcoming termination. My comments may make it even more difficult for Sallie to explore any mixed feelings she has about my news. Her comments become even more distant.

It is rare for a patient to be able to process her feelings about a termination immediately. This is one of the reasons we recommend announcing the termination date far ahead of time. After a while, Sallie may be able to express fear, anger, or sadness about the upcoming parting. My job is to tolerate whatever emotions she is experiencing at the moment and to help her to understand her feelings—and the defenses against them.

EXAMPLE 17.2A (the Indifferent Patient)

The therapist announces that she will be leaving the city in 6 months and listens carefully to her patient's reactions

15 Minutes into the Session

THERAPIST: I have some news I need to tell you today.

SALLIE: Oh, what?

THERAPIST: Well, in July I will be moving out of Boston.

SALLIE: So I won't be able to see you anymore?

THERAPIST: That's true. Our work together will need to end before I leave.

SALLIE: Oh, okay. (*nonchalance*) So when is your last week here exactly?

THERAPIST: I will be leaving the last week in June.

SALLIE: Where are you going?

THERAPIST: I will be moving to Florida. But I know this unexpected news affects our work together. What is it like to hear it?

SALLIE: Oh, I don't care that much. People move on. I can see someone else at the clinic, can't I?

THERAPIST: Yes, if you wish. I can set you up with a referral to continue therapy after I leave. (*Nods encouragingly.*)

SALLIE: Okay, that's fine. One therapist is as good as another, I guess.

THERAPIST: [*I wait quietly, but I don't nod in agreement to Sallie's last comment. I remember that my supervisors predicted that some patients would respond to my announcement with nonchalance, and I try not to take Sallie's response personally. While I feel hurt that Sallie, a patient I have enjoyed working with, is reacting this way, I try to listen carefully to her next association.*]

SALLIE: I'm not a big fan of endings so I just ignore them.

THERAPIST: How do you ignore them? [*This is an interesting lead.*]

SALLIE: I just don't think about them at all. It makes it easier than getting all choked up.

THERAPIST: Choked up isn't easy.

SALLIE: No, of course, it sucks. I don't want to think about it. I'd rather tell you about the latest stuff at school.

THERAPIST: Okay. We can leave this for now. Maybe we can talk about it some more another time.

EXAMPLE 17.2B (the Upset Patient)

15 Minutes into the Session

THERAPIST: I have some news I need to tell you today.

SALLIE: Oh, what?

THERAPIST: Well, in July I will be leaving Boston.

SALLIE: You will—*what*?!

THERAPIST: (*sensitive look*) I will only be working in the clinic until June 30th.

SALLIE: That is horrible news! I can't believe it—and I was just beginning to feel comfortable working with you. Where are you going?

THERAPIST: I will be moving to Florida.

SALLIE: Well, that is fine and nice for you, I guess. I'm glad one of us will be happy, while I continue to struggle along here in "balmy" Boston.

THERAPIST: [*I notice but don't react outwardly to the sarcasm in the previous comment.*] It's difficult news for you to hear.

SALLIE: It's horrible. You know, I was just starting to think that maybe you cared about our work together. I guess I was wrong about that one.

THERAPIST: As I am leaving you at a sensitive time, it feels like I don't care about you.

SALLIE: That's right. (*Starts to cry.*) I don't know what to do now.

THERAPIST: [*I sit quietly with Sallie crying for a few moments.*]

SALLIE: So now what?

THERAPIST: Could you share with me the words behind the tears?

SALLIE: I don't know. Nothing and everything, I guess.

THERAPIST: It makes sense that news that I'll be leaving brings up a whole host of feelings. I do want to hear about them.

SALLIE: Whatever. I just feel in shock right now.

THERAPIST: What do you mean when you say "shock?"

SALLIE: I don't want to think about it anymore. I think I'll go to the gym and work out.

THERAPIST: Separations, especially when they are a surprise, can feel shocking.

Examples 17.2A and 17.2B illustrate two common reactions in response to an unexpected termination date: an emotional withdrawal or an intense expression of feeling. In the withdrawal example (17.2A), I tolerate my own distress at Sallie's indifference. Then, I learn that Sallie's attitude is her *modus operandi* when faced with a sad good-bye. In Example 17.2B, I avoid diminishing Sallie's intense reaction to my news and try to affirm it instead. Since some patients react self-injuriously to an impending loss of a therapist, I gently asked Sallie what it means for her to "feel in shock." Her response is reassuringly healthy and adaptive.

In both cases, I do not push Sallie to delve deeply into her feelings right after my announcement. There will be plenty of time to discuss her reaction in more detail during future sessions.

A PATIENT'S DECOMPENSATION
CENTERED ON TERMINATION

Once I set the date of the last session with a patient, I can anticipate a variety of responses during the process of saying good-bye.

Some patients may start flooding each remaining session with a barrage of new material, pushing themselves to discuss previously avoided problems in view of the new time limitation.

Others may have more trouble with the impending separation. Patients who were always on time may start coming late to sessions or missing them altogether. Others may become more openly hostile as the date of the last session approaches. For them, it might be easier to leave in an angry state rather than to work through the sadness of ending.

Patients with a fragile adaptive capacity and a limited support system outside of therapy may be at risk for an increase in regressed behavior or even a decompensation. A previously stable patient may stop taking her medications and become morose, depressed, and even suicidal. If the termination has been announced months in advance, there may be ample time to work through the crises before our final meeting.

Whatever the instigating stressor, preserving the patient's safety is always the first priority at any stage of treatment. As the termination date approaches, patients who need increased emotional support can access additional treatment via self-help or therapeutic groups, psychopharmacological consultations, adjustments of medications, or contacts with appropriate religious or social organizations. If the patient's safety is at risk, a day program or an emergency hospitalization during the termination period may become necessary. (For more details on how to help a suicidal patient, see Chapter 9.)

I might handpick the new therapist who will take my place for patients who need to continue treatment without a break. Overlapping my last sessions with the first few consultation sessions with the new therapist can be immensely comforting to a patient who relies on therapy to support her everyday functioning.

In Example 17.3, Candice Jones has trouble coping with our upcoming termination.

EXAMPLE 17.3

The patient decompensates after the therapist announces the date that treatment will end

CANDICE: Dr. Bender, since you told me that you were going to leave, I have been feeling very odd. I haven't slept well at all the past couple of weeks. (*Starts to cry.*) Now and then, I feel as bad as I did when we first met!

THERAPIST: It sounds like you have really been suffering.

CANDICE: Sometimes I don't even know if it is worth continuing the struggle. I know I will feel so lost without our sessions. I don't know what will happen to me. (*Grabs for many tissues.*)

THERAPIST: Have you been thinking of death?

CANDICE: Now and then. Yes, to tell you the truth, I have. I feel so lost. I'm not sure where to turn.

I complete a thorough evaluation of suicidal risk as outlined in Chapter 9. Candice's actual risk of hurting herself is very low.

THERAPIST: Feeling lost after you had been feeling better is very distressing. Let's think together how to provide what you need so you can weather this tough time safely. [*I take a supportive, problem-solving, cognitive stance because Candice is already overwhelmed by her feelings.*]

CANDICE: I need *you*, Dr. Bender, not a baby-sitting plan. Therapy helps me manage.

THERAPIST: It is not easy to lose a therapist. I know it doesn't take the pain away, but I do want you to know that I have a great deal of trust in Dr. Powell. I feel confident that she will be able to help you during this transition time. [*Dr. Powell is the new therapist I have found for Candice.*]

CANDICE: That helps a little bit, but you know that it is incredibly difficult to start working with someone new. (*Sniffs.*)

THERAPIST: It is difficult.

CANDICE: Yes, and I still feel overwhelmed.

THERAPIST: It is troubling news that I will be leaving and that you will have to start anew.

Right now, it may be difficult to recognize the progress you have made since we started working together. Over the months to come, you and I will have time to plan for the extra support that you might need.

In Example 17.3, Candice has trouble coping with her conflicting feelings of dismay, yearning, and anger that she feels about our parting. She regresses, losing the ability to calm herself and falls back on old faulty coping mechanisms. To shore up Candice's more mature adaptations, I employ a cognitive approach. She will also do better during this stressful time with additional therapeutic supports that attempt to minimize regression and to maximize adaptive psychological functioning.

THE PATIENT SETS THE TERMINATION DATE

Patients end therapy in a variety of ways. There is a large group of people who never truly terminate because they prefer to drop in for intermittent therapy sessions ("tune-ups," as some patients have called them) depending on their need. When this group of patients starts to feel better, they often taper their session frequency (for instance, from once a week to once a month.)

Sometimes, a patient will plan a longer break away from treatment without scheduling a future session. While I'll let the patient know that I will welcome her return, I can't guarantee that a weekly spot will be immediately available if she wishes to resume at this frequency. I can usually fit intermittent as-needed sessions into my schedule with some notice. While a break for a number of months isn't a true termination, I'll encourage a review of the therapy in the little time we have left before the separation.

Premature terminations (often necessitated by a geographical move) or mature terminations are more definite. Interestingly enough, similar psychodynamic issues emerge whether the therapist or the patient initiates the termination.

SALLIE GANE'S TERMINATION

In order to discuss termination issues in Sallie Gane's therapy, we need to fast-forward her treatment past the transference discussions that began in Chapter 16. To resolve her emotional conflicts about her career and family, many more sessions would need to follow, focusing on Sallie's difficulties with her female peers and with her mother. During this process, I could continue to use information gleaned from the transference to increase our understanding of these issues.

This process could be very slow. Psychodynamic psychotherapy is not a microwaveable process; it cooks along more like a crockpot. In order for Sallie to sustain long-term emotional change, her core emotional issues would need to be examined jointly multiple times from many different perspectives. (In the psychodynamic literature, this process is known as working through.)

Both the experience of feeling validated and the increased understanding of her conflicts and motivations will be therapeutic for Sallie. She will gain insight that her controlling behavior toward Charlie was an identification with her mother. With this awareness, she may choose to behave differently in future relationships. Slowly, she may foster friendships with people, like Emme, who appreciate and support her strengths and individuality, unlike Gwen.

Eventually, Sallie might gather the courage to plot her own career course and to discuss this plan with her mother. We'll say she decides to pursue journalism as a profession after all. After completing her college courses and finishing her therapy with me, she decides to move to New York City to start her graduate studies. Again, remember that every sentence in this paragraph reflects hours of therapy, using many of the techniques outlined in our previous chapters.

Eventually, the time to say good-bye would approach. Our termination would become another therapeutic opportunity. As we review our work together, we'll discuss aspects of the therapy that have been helpful as well as those that have been disappointing. Again, even in its ending, therapy can model a relationship that is resilient enough to weather constructive criticisms as well as compliments.

In Example 17.4, Sallie announces her upcoming move to New York to pursue graduate school in her chosen profession. This vignette also illustrates another typical termination pattern—when a patient copes with an upcoming termination by ignoring it. Even though it may feel easier to collude with this process, it is my responsibility to refocus the treatment intermittently on our impending separation.

EXAMPLE 17.4

The patient announces her forthcoming move and then tries to ignore the upcoming separation from the therapist

SALLIE: (*In April*) Dr. Bender, I have amazing news!

THERAPIST: Let's hear it!

SALLIE: Well, you know how we have talked *ad nauseum* about the fact I am more interested in journalism than business? And, you know how we talked about how my mother was surprised to learn this but was not anywhere near as upset as I had imagined?

THERAPIST: Yes. (*Nods encouragingly.*)

SALLIE: Well, I didn't tell you this because it felt sort of scary, but after one of our sessions I filled out an application to a university in New York that has a great journalism department. The only people who knew about it were the teachers I needed to ask for letters of recommendation. It felt like such a gamble. I didn't want to let people know, because I didn't think my chances of getting in were very good.

Umm, well, guess what? I'm in! I can't believe it. They took me! I just received my acceptance letter this morning. After I graduate this spring, I'll need to move to New York City right away to get settled. That is if I am brave enough to go through with this. I can't believe it.

THERAPIST: (*supportive tone and smiling*) Why not? This is very exciting news. What do you think you want to do?

SALLIE: I think I might do it. It just sounds so amazing. But, I keep pinching myself. I can't believe this is happening to me!

As the weeks progress, Sallie relates her plans to move to New York but does not mention anything about the impending termination. She almost acts as if I will be moving away with her.

SALLIE: So I am leaving Boston July 15th and starting at my new school on the first of September. I have so much to do. I need to find housing. I need to find a roommate. (*Eyes widen.*) It still doesn't feel real.

THERAPIST: And we will be saying good-bye.

SALLIE: Well, maybe I'll stay in Boston until late August, so we won't have to stop for a few more months.

THERAPIST: What will it feel like to stop meeting?

SALLIE: Oh, I am just trying to ignore it.

THERAPIST: Is there a way that I can help you to notice it?

SALLIE: What do you mean?

THERAPIST: Well, I think it is important for us to talk about the fact that our work together will be ending.

SALLIE: Why?

THERAPIST: I think the ending of our meetings is an important part of the therapy. It can solidify what we've worked on together. Also, learning how to say good-bye in a meaningful way is a skill in itself.

SALLIE: Well, if I don't say good-bye, it doesn't feel as complete or as sad. It's more like a "see-you-later."

THERAPIST: "See-you-laters" are easier than complete good-byes?

SALLIE: Yes, I'll really miss you, and I just don't want to think about it.

THERAPIST: Can you tell me what is hard about thinking about it?

SALLIE: I feel so excited to be doing something just for me. This is what we have talked about for months. You know, following my dream, not my mother's. But it is also scary to be ending therapy. You've been a really important person in my life. I don't like to think about giving you up. It makes me nervous.

THERAPIST: The nervous part detracts from the exciting part. Maybe if we talk about it together, you may feel a little less nervous.

SALLIE: I doubt it. I'd rather just ignore it for now. It feels to weird to say good-bye to you forever. What if I get to New York and freak out? I just get scared thinking about it.

THERAPIST: Maybe it would be useful to think about how I could be most supportive of the move. If it would help, we could touch base by phone, or even schedule a phone session as you get settled in New York. If you would like to continue psychotherapy in New York, I can try to help you find a new therapist.

SALLIE: That does make me feel better. The idea of never talking to you again is scary to me.

THERAPIST: After we've worked together so closely, it can feel scary to end our weekly meetings, and I hope we can talk more about this. But, I'm still interested in your well-being, and would be happy to touch base by phone, as I mentioned.

If Sallie tries to ignore our impending separation, it is my responsibility to remind her gently, fairly often, of how many sessions we have left. If the ending of therapy is dealt with in an honest, direct, and genuine manner, Sallie might be able to use this experience to strengthen her ability to cope with other separations throughout her life. Morbid or pathological grief reactions may be partially due to unresolved partings, so an increased ability to process good-byes may even prevent future psychological distress.

Brief phone conversations or a few scheduled phone sessions may be a great support to Sallie during her transition. I try to balance my offer of phone availability with a continued focus on the ending of the face-to-face weekly treatment.

THE PATIENT WHO DISAPPEARS AS THE TERMINATION APPROACHES

Now and then, a patient might feel so threatened by the upcoming loss that she may stop attending sessions weeks before the termination date.

Because it can be so easy to under- or overreact when a patient disappears, it is useful to have a protocol in place for this type of situation. (See Chapter 10 for more details.)

If Sallie unexpectedly missed a session as her termination date approached, I would call her at a time that I expected her to be at home. If I am unable to talk to her directly, I might leave the following message, worded carefully to preserve confidentiality: "Hello, this is Suzanne Bender calling for Sallie Gane. I was concerned when I did not see you at your scheduled appointment today. Please call me to confirm our appointment for next week at our regular time."

This message encourages Sallie to be in touch with me regardless of whether she plans to return for her next appointment. Sometimes after one missed session a patient will return to her regularly scheduled session without difficulty. We'll then have ample time to discuss the upcoming termination. Other times the first missed session might be a harbinger of repeated absences with numerous excuses, all in preparation for our future separation.

In response to Sallie's hypothetical disappearance, I would follow my billing protocol for last-minute cancellations or missed sessions. (Please see Chapters 8 and 10 for more details.) I might also consider writing a letter inviting her back to treatment. (See Figure 17.1.)

If Sallie returns to treatment after she receives my letter, I will ad-

---

[Professional letterhead]

Date

Sallie Gane's address

Dear Ms. Sallie Gane:

I am sorry that I have not received a response from you since our last phone call on April 8th. Since I have not heard from you, I do not know how you are doing, but I hope you are doing well.

I am still available to meet with you to conclude our work together before you leave. I hope that we shall have this opportunity. If I do not see you before you leave, I want you to know that I wish you the best. If you desire to schedule a meeting any time in the future, please feel free to call me.

Sincerely,

Suzanne Bender MD
My office phone numbers

FIGURE 17.1. Letter inviting the patient to return to treatment.

dress her repeated absences midway through our reunion meeting. As Sallie's disappearance obviously endangers the possibility of a thoughtful termination, it deserves immediate attention.

It's possible that Sallie may deny that her repeated missed sessions have any emotional meaning. If so, there isn't much I can do but follow her lead. Termination is like every other part of therapy. The treatment proceeds at the patient's pace. Topics can be introduced, but forcing the discussion will rarely produce any useful results.

A PATIENT EXPRESSES HER APPRECIATION DURING THE TERMINATION

Interestingly enough, sometimes a patient can be better at expressing her gratitude at the end of treatment than a therapist may be at accepting it. I was caught off guard the first time a patient sincerely expressed how much I had helped her and how much she would miss me. I had to learn how to acknowledge a patient's compliments just as I had to learn how to listen to her complaints.

While it isn't useful for me to lead with my own feelings about a termination, I have an opportunity to share my own feelings when a patient expresses her appreciation.

EXAMPLE 17.5

The patient expresses her gratitude toward her therapist, and the therapist responds

SALLIE: So today is our last session.

THERAPIST: Yes.

SALLIE: I'll really miss you.

THERAPIST: I will miss you too.

SALLIE: (*Smiles.*) That is so nice to hear. I know you aren't supposed to feel connected to your patients or anything. Rules of the trade, I guess.

THERAPIST: Does it feel like I couldn't feel connected to you because of the rules of the therapy?

SALLIE: Sort of. You have so many patients. I can't imagine that I mean something special.

THERAPIST: Why not?

SALLIE: I don't know. I don't want to set myself up for disappointment. Anyway, I have learned so much in here. It has been a good experience.

THERAPIST: I have learned as well. I admired seeing how you mastered many of your difficulties with your mother and found a new group of friends who are more supportive.

SALLIE: Really?

THERAPIST: Really.

SALLIE: That is so nice. The therapy actually really helped me. There were times I was sure my life would never improve, but in fact, it really has.

THERAPIST: You have worked very hard. It has been very gratifying for me to be a part of this process.

SALLIE: Wow. It really means so much to hear you say that.

THERAPIST: It comes as a surprise?

SALLIE: I just never imagined that I was affecting you as well.

THERAPIST: Any idea why not?

SALLIE: I never felt that important.

THERAPIST: How do you feel to hear that you are?

SALLIE: Scared, but really happy also.

THERAPIST: Scared?

SALLIE: I don't want to do anything wrong to disappoint you. I'm not perfect, you know.

THERAPIST: Do you feel that I'll be disappointed if you are not perfect?

SALLIE: A little bit. I don't want to mess it up. I don't know. I still feel this way sometimes with friends too. You know, same old thing.

THERAPIST: You have an increased awareness and understanding about it, but it still might feel like a lot of pressure for you to endure.

SALLIE: Yeah, I guess it is.

THERAPIST: (Nods.)

SALLIE: I'm sorry that I can't just savor our last meeting, and we have to talk about this uncomfortable stuff.

THERAPIST: It feels like you've used up your time to talk about more uncomfortable stuff? (empathic look)

SALLIE: Maybe.(*Smiles.*)

THERAPIST: It can be difficult to say good-bye when there are issues that remain that you would have liked to work on. [*I had mentioned in previous meetings that Sallie could always seek further therapy in New York if she thinks it could be useful. During our last session I keep the focus on Sallie and me rather than punting the issue to a future therapist.*]

SALLIE: Exactly! I'll really miss how you make things feel okay instead of overwhelming.

THERAPIST: We have done good work together, and it makes sense that it feels hard to stop.

SALLIE: If I ever move back to Boston, can I give you a call or set up a special session?

THERAPIST: Sure, I would be glad to know how you are doing.

SALLIE: Okay. That makes me feel better. I guess it is time to stop now.

THERAPIST: It is.

SALLIE: (*Stands up.*) Thanks for everything.

THERAPIST: You are very welcome. I wish you the best.

In Example 17.5, Sallie and I express our mutual appreciation for one another. The parting is sweet and sour, as many are. While Sallie recognizes how much she has grown during the therapy, she can also identify some remaining issues that might require future attention. She may also be bringing up these difficulties in the final session as a way of reconnecting with me before she leaves. With this possibility in mind, I do not jump to refer Sallie to a therapist in New York for work on these remaining issues but instead keep the focus on our separation.

Is a termination forever? Historically, terminations were viewed as permanent endings. Once a patient had finished psychoanalysis, for instance, it was not considered therapeutic, by some analysts, for the patient to return to treatment even if she ran into future emotional difficulties. Since then, therapists' views have become more flexible. While it is important to view a therapy's termination as a completion of a piece of work, this does not mean that future meetings cannot occur. While therapists who are ending practice, moving, or finishing training are notable exceptions, many clinicians explicitly invite their patients to call them in the future. It might be helpful to meet again if setbacks occur or to report progress or further success.

Sallie may leave for New York to attend journalism school but then return to Boston the following summer and request a few sessions. It doesn't make sense to refuse her these sessions merely because she terminated a year earlier. It might be fruitful for Sallie to meet for a short time, if only to review her experience during the academic year. Because I know Sallie so well, the therapy can carry on rather nicely once she has filled me in on the recent details. It is also possible that Sallie may move back to Boston when her education is completed. She may wish to get some help with a subsequent phase of her development. Again, leaving the door open for future work can be highly beneficial.

What if Sallie is seeing a new therapist in New York but spends the summer in Boston and calls to see me for a few sessions? Should I see Sallie even if she is in formal treatment with someone else in New York? This dilemma should be approached gingerly, trying to keep Sallie's best interests in mind. It might be best if she could schedule phone sessions with her current therapist in New York. If this isn't possible (for example, if the therapist is on vacation), I could serve as the interim therapist. It wouldn't be right to leave Sallie without any treatment, especially if her problem is urgent.

Having two therapists might feel confusing to Sallie, so my very limited treatment of Sallie should address her current distress while supporting her resumption of treatment in New York at the end of the summer. Involving the therapist in New York in the treatment plan would help Sallie reconnect with her local clinician when she returns.

Therapy is an exceptional experience in many ways. While the therapist and patient work together closely, the ultimate goal is for the patient to complete the work and to end the relationship. A therapist must play successive roles: being available to the patient during therapy and being ready and willing to support the patient's leaving when the treatment is over.

Inner strength and equanimity combined with an emotionally fulfilling life can help a therapist weather the partings with her patients. Knowing oneself and connecting with family and friends reduce the likelihood of the therapist clinging to her patients emotionally.

Meanwhile, with each ending of therapy, I learn something new about myself. Partings with people we care about are experiences we work on throughout our lives and not always with as much forethought and autognosis as we bring to the therapeutic encounter. The more we can be in touch with the feelings that emerge in separations, the more we will mature as people and as therapists.

Key words: artificial termination, bereavement, decompensation, forced termination, grief reaction, interruption of therapy, maturation, mature termination, natural termination, psychotherapy, regression, separations, separation anxiety, termination, therapeutic alliance, therapeutic goal, working through

Epilogue

The field of mental health continues to advance and to expand. With new developments in psychopharmacology, neuroscience, and neuroimaging, we have a deeper understanding of the interaction between human biology and psychology. Innovative treatments are producing huge benefits for suffering patients. But no matter how much we discover about brain function, it can never replace the power of understanding and being understood. The work of a psychotherapist is unique and will be needed for the imaginable future.

The journey to become a psychotherapist is complicated but enriching. While the beginning of training may feel challenging, over time, the confusion abates, and it becomes clear how to conduct a treatment. Eventually, the trainee realizes that she knows enough to start, continue, and end a treatment independently. Equally important, she knows when and where to access help if she needs it.

We have tried to impart the skills that beginning therapists will need to practice effectively. Use them with compassion—for your patients and for yourselves.

Glossary

ADD   Attention-deficit disorder: The former and now obsolete name for attention-deficit/hyperactivity disorder (ADHD).

ADHD   Attention-deficit/hyperactivity disorder: A persistent condition that begins prior to age 7 and that causes impairment in functioning at home and at school or at work through patterns of inattention and/or hyperactivity and/or impulsivity.

Adjustment disorder   A condition that involves impairment of social, occupational, or academic functioning with symptoms that arise within 3 months of one or more recognizable psychosocial stressors.

Affect   The outward expression of emotion through vocalization, facial expression, or other nonverbal behavior.

Affective equivalent   A symptom that substitutes for an emotional expression, for example, a pain in the neck (or elsewhere).

Agoraphobia   An irrational dread of open spaces or public places.

Alliance, therapeutic   The collaboration between a patient and a clinician intended to accomplish the goal(s) of treatment.

Anorexia nervosa   An eating disorder that features voluntary reduction of food intake to keep well below (85% or less) expected body weight.

Association   A word, thought, image, feeling, or other experience that arises spontaneously in response to an internal or external stimulus.

Association, free   An association that arises without either internal or external prompting.

Autognosis   Knowledge, with understanding, of one's self.

Automatic thoughts   Ideas that arise without conscious intention or control.

Autonomy   Independence, freedom from external control.

Axes I–V   Five categories of information employed by clinicians to design a treatment program appropriate for each patient. This approach is advocated by DSM-IV.

Axis I: Psychiatric disorders or problems.
Axis II: Disorders of personality or mental retardation.
Axis III: Medical conditions or problems.
Axis IV: Problems in the patient's psychosocial and environmental aspects of the patient's life.
Axis V: An estimate of how well the patient functions.

Blank slate   A metaphor often used to describe therapists who disclose little about themselves in order to permit freer fantasies and transferences by their patients.

Boundary   The limit to personal or social contact between clinician and patient.

Bulimia nervosa   An eating disorder that features a pattern of food intake in binges and followed by efforts to compensate with self-induced vomiting, intestinal purging, or other means in an attempt to keep weight from rising.

Cardiac dysrhythmia   Irregular heartbeat.

Chief complaint   The main symptom or problem that a patient reports to a clinician.

Clarification   An explanation by the therapist intended to enlarge the patient's understanding of current subject matter. It does not necessarily include a historical or developmental perspective.

Cognitive-behavioral therapy   A form of psychosocial treatment based on the relearning of beliefs, concepts, attitudes, and/or actions.

Cognitive restructuring   The process of altering a subject's beliefs, attitudes, expectations, or concepts about her experiences.

Comorbid   The relationship between two or more disorders that afflict a person at the same time.

Confidentiality   The secrecy of information revealed to a mental health clinician that is protected by ethical principles and law.

Conflict   Mutual opposition, usually referring to wishes, goals, or purposes.

Confrontation   The process in which a clinician calls the patient's attention to ideas or other information.

Conscious memory   *See* Evocative memory.

Consent, informed   Permission regarding an offered procedure given by a patient, without coercion, and based on adequate knowledge of benefits, risks, costs, duration, and other factors.

Contract   An agreement, usually spoken although sometimes written, between a patient and a clinician, about specific behaviors related to a treatment. For example, a patient may promise to call the clinician or to go to the nearest emergency room when suicidal intentions increase, as a contract for safety.

Contraindication   A factor or circumstance that makes a particular treatment or procedure undesirable or fraught with unnecessary danger.

Counterresistance   Behavior by the clinician, usually outside her awareness, that opposes the progress of treatment.

Countertransference   Subjective responses of a clinician toward a patient.

Countertransference enactment   Expression of feelings or attitudes of the therapist in response to the patient, which are partly or wholly outside of consciousness.

Crisis, developmental   A time in a person's life in which her role changes markedly, such as puberty, marriage, parenthood.

Crisis, normative   Situations or events that commonly occur in human lives which lead to substantial role changes, such as the death of a loved one, loss of a job, promotions, injuries, and so on.

Day residue   Portions of recent experiences that appear in a dream.

DSM-IV   The *Diagnostic and Statistical Manual of Mental Disorders*, fourth edition (see the entry in the Bibliography.), a detailed and descriptive catalogue of mental disorders generally accepted as authoritative in the United States, Canada, and other countries.

Duty to report   A legal requirement,which overrides confidentiality, that a clinician inform governmental authorities when she learns of such matters as current or intended abuse of children, the disabled, or the elderly. Duties vary among jurisdictions.

Dysphoria   An unpleasant emotional state.

Eating disorder   A condition in which behavior related to eating is so extreme that it interferes seriously with personal or occupational functioning, and endangers health.

Ego boundary   The mental function that enables a person to distinguish between stimuli that originate outside herself from those that originate inside herself, for example, the ability to distinguish between an actual voice and a hallucination.

Electroconvulsive Therapy (ECT)   The use of a weak electric current applied to the sides of a patient's head (bilateral) or to one side and the top of her head (unilateral). This treatment is offered to patients suffering from disorders such as severe depression or mania, usually after multiple trials of medication have not provided relief. The treatment is conducted with brief general anesthesia aided by muscle relaxants under the care of a trained anesthesiologist with full resuscitation equipment.

Empathic lapse   A misunderstanding of the patient by the therapist (*see also* Empathy).

Empathy   The attempt to recognize another person's subjective state cognitively and/or emotionally.

Enactment   The interpersonal expression, through speech or movement, of ideas, emotions, attitudes, or other internal (intrapsychic) experiences.

Ethics   Considerations of what is good or bad, right or wrong, acceptable or unacceptable in human behavior.

Evocative memory   The ability to call up or to bring to consciousness an event, image, or experience as desired. Also known as explicit memory or conscious memory.

Explicit memory   *See* Evocative memory.

Extraparietal   Outside the walls (of the office, clinic, or hospital).

Fantasy   That which is imagined.

Fantasy, directed   Something that is imagined intentionally, with a purpose or design.

Fiduciary   Someone who is entrusted with power for the benefit of someone else.

Formulation   A systematic appraisal of an individual's biopsychosocial condition, often including hypotheses about its development and about how to improve it.

Frame   The limits or boundaries of the relationship in which psychotherapy is conducted.

Generalized anxiety disorder   Worry and anxiety that are difficult to control, for a majority of days over a period of 6 months or more, that cause significant distress and impairment of functioning in social, occupational, or other important areas.

Genogram   A diagram of a family tree.

Group psychotherapy   Any form of psychosocial treatment in which a therapist or leader works with more than one patient.

Hatred   Extreme hostility.

Here and now   The current relationship of the therapist and the patient.

Hostility   An attitude of antagonism or animosity. It is like hatred if it includes a desire to do harm. Its emotional quality tends to last longer than anger.

Iatrogenic   Caused by a physician (or other health care professional or institution).

Idealization   A defensive process in which someone or something is thought of as perfect or as having extremely favorable qualities.

Ideas of reference   A belief that one is the object of special attention, messages, or meaning. For example, someone named Tom might see a sign with the letter "T" advertising the public transportation system and believe it is a message meant for him individually.

Identification   A process by which a person believes or assumes that she has the qualities or features of someone else. The person may be aware to some extent of this process.

Identification, complementary   The experience by the therapist of emotions and/or attitudes similar to those experienced by significant people in the patient's personal life.

Identification, concurrent   The experience by the therapist of emotions and/or attitudes similar to those experienced by the patient.

Imagery   A mental likeness of a person, place, situation, or story, actual or fanciful.

Imagery, directed   A mental likeness of a person, place, situation, or story, actual or fanciful, created with a conscious purpose.

Impasse   A position from which there is, or appears to be, no way out; a deadlock or a dilemma.

Insight   Understanding one's emotional processes and experiences with a combination of feelings and intellect.

Interpretation   An explanation offered by a therapist to help the patient understand her inner experience in a way that includes her feelings as well as thoughts, and that links her experiences in the past with those in the present.

Intersubjectivity   The effects that the emotional experience and attitudes of the patient have on the emotional experience and attitudes of the therapist and vice versa.

Latency   The period of a child's life from about the age of 5 or 6 until the onset of puberty.

Learning disability   A condition in which a child of average or above average intelligence experiences specific difficulty in learning (*see also* Learning disorder).

Learning disorder   The term used in DSM-IV to signify learning disability.

Litigation   A lawsuit and its related procedures.

Mania   A condition characterized by elevated or irritable mood, persisting for at least 1 week, accompanied by at least three of the following: decreased need for sleep, flight of ideas, tangential and/or pressured speech, increased pleasurable activity, motor agitation, and others. It is sometimes accompanied by psychosis. It must interfere with social or occupational functioning.

Manipulation   The process of influencing someone, often without that person's awareness of what, how, or why it is being done.

Mentor   A trusted advisor and educator.

Mood   Emotion felt inwardly.

Narcissistic injury   An insult to someone's pride.

Neurochemistry   The science that deals with properties and interactions of substances important to the nervous system.

Neuropsychiatry   The medical subspecialty that deals with mental and emotional disorders and their relationship with the nervous system.

Neurotransmitters   Chemical substances that mediate communication between nerve cells.

Neurovegetative   Refers to basic life functions controlled by the nervous system such as appetite, sleep, energy, and motion.

Objectivity   A condition of being unbiased and not affected by one's personal feelings, attitudes, or goals.

Osteoporosis   A condition in which the density of bones, and therefore their strength, is reduced and the possibility of fractures is increased. Patients suffering from anorexia nervosa complicated by amenorrhea are at risk for this condition.

Peer supervision   Mutual teaching and learning between colleagues.

Personal therapy   Psychosocial treatment, including psychoanalysis, undergone by a trainee or a graduate clinician.

Personality disorder   A condition consisting of a lasting set of inner experiences and outward behaviors that impair social, occupational or academic function or that produce intense subjective distress. It begins in early adulthood and tends to be inflexible.

Posttraumatic stress disorder (PTSD)   A condition persisting for more than 1 month with symptoms such as recurrently distressing recollections, hypervigilance, avoidance, startle responses, nightmares, or emotional dulling, following an event in which the patient experienced horror and helplessness when exposed to a threat of death, to dire injury to oneself, or to the death or mutilation of others.

Privileged communication   Information provided by a patient to a clinician which must be kept secret, in accordance with laws and ethical principles, unless the patient authorizes disclosure.

Process notes   Records kept by a clinician that can include descriptions of interactions and nonverbal communications as well as the clinician's reactions and perceptions.

Psychoeducation   Teaching about mental, emotional, or interpersonal conditions or disorders.

Psychological review of systems   A series of questions posed by a clinician to a patient about the possible presence of symptoms related to the main categories of mental disorders such as anxiety disorders, mood disorders, substance-related disorders, psychotic disorders, and others.

Psychomotor agitation   Excessive motion that is unproductive, tends to be repetitive, and is accompanied by inner feelings of tension.

Psychomotor retardation   A general slowing of motion and speech often accompanied by apathy or unhappy mood.

Psychopathology   The study of mental disorders based on scientific research. Often used to refer to mental abnormality.

Psychopharmacology   A subspecialty of medicine that deals with medications for mental and emotional disorders.

Psychotherapy   Any treatment of a mental or emotional disorder that relies on communication between patient(s) and clinician(s) without the use of medicine.

Psychotropic   Mind-affecting. Commonly refers to drugs, both legal and illegal.

Rapport   A harmonious mutually accepting relationship between two people.

Reliability   The consistency with which a test or other measuring method will show closely similar results when employed repeatedly under similar conditions.

Repetition compulsion   The impulse to reenact previous developmental experiences with people in one's current life.

Resistance   Any behavior over which the patient has some influence that interferes with the progress of treatment.

Reversal of roles   A situation in which a person, who is under the care of another, is induced to provide care to the original caretaker.

Review of systems   A series of questions posed by a clinician to a patient about the possible presence of symptoms related to the major physiological systems, such as the cardiovascular, respiratory, gastrointestinal, neurological, and others.

Sadism   Pleasure or enjoyment in inflicting suffering.

Subpoena   A document that summons witnesses, documents, or other evidence before a court or other official body.

Supportive intervention   A procedure in psychotherapy in which the clinician reinforces the patient's most adaptive coping mechanisms or introduces more effective ones.

Stalking   Pursuing someone in a predatory manner. Unwelcome, threatening, intimidating contacts or communications persisting despite the quarry's wishes.

Termination   The ending phase of treatment.

Thought broadcasting   A belief or subjective experience that one's thoughts are converted into sound and can be heard by others.

Thought insertion   A belief or subjective experience that others can put thoughts into one's mind. The "inserted" thoughts are experienced as not one's own.

Transference   The conveyance of feelings, attitudes, yearnings, or ideas about one person to another person. A patient may transfer feelings or attitudes toward a parent to the therapist.

Validity   The degree to which a test or other measuring method truly measures what it is claimed to measure. For example, an intelligence test printed in Japanese administered to subjects who can read only English would have extremely low validity, because correct answers would occur only by chance (random guessing).

Working through   A process, which leads to insight, based upon a person's examination of her problems multiple times and from various points of view.

Bibliography

Alonso A, Swiller H. *Group Therapy in Clinical Practice.* Washington, DC: American Psychiatric Press, 1993.

American Medical Association. *Current Procedural Terminology (CPT).* Chicago: American Medical Association, 2001.

American Psychiatric Association. *Diagnostic and Statistical Manual of Mental Disorders, Fourth Edition.* Washington, DC: American Psychiatric Association, 1994.

Anfang SA, Appelbaum PS. Twenty years after Tarasoff: Reviewing the duty to protect. *Harvard Review of Psychiatry* 1996; 4: 67–76.

Basch MF. *Doing Psychotherapy.* New York: Basic Books, 1980.

Beck JS. *Cognitive Therapy: Basics and Beyond.* New York: Guilford Press, 1995.

Bibring E. Psychoanalysis and the dynamic psychotherapies. *Journal of the American Psychoanalytic Association* 1954; 2: 745–70.

Bremner JD. Does stress damage the brain? *Biological Psychiatry* 1999; 45(7): 797–805. (Review)

Bromfield R. *Doing Child and Adolescent Psychotherapy: The Ways and Whys.* Northvale, NJ: Jason Aronson, 1999.

Bruch H. *Learning Psychotherapy: Rationale and Ground Rules.* Cambridge, MA: Harvard University Press, 1974.

Ciraulo DA, Shader RI, eds. *Clinical Manual of Chemical Dependency.* Washington, DC: American Psychiatric Press, 1991.

Ewing JA. Detecting alcoholism: The CAGE questionnaire. *Journal of the American Medical Association* 1984; 252: 1905–1907.

Faber A, Mazlish E. *How to Talk So Kids Will Listen and Listen So Kids Will Talk.* New York: Avon Books, 1980. (A clear book that teaches empathic listening.)

Falk WE. *DIG FAST: A mnemonic for mania.* Presentation, MGH postgraduate course: Psychopharmacology, Boston, personal communication, 1984.

Fraiberg, S. *The Magic Years: Understanding and Handling the Problems of Early Childhood.* New York: Scribner, 1959.

Gaylin W. *Talk Is Not Enough: How Psychotherapy Really Works*. Boston: Little, Brown, 2000.

Gutheil TG, Gabbard GO. Misuses and misunderstandings of boundary theory in clinical and regulatory settings. *American Journal of Psychiatry* 1998; 155: 409–14.

Hales RE, Yudofsky SC, Talbott JA, eds. *Textbook of Psychiatry*, 3rd ed. Washington DC: American Psychiatric Press, 1999.

Hirschfeld RMA, Russell JM. Assessment and treatment of suicidal patients. *New England Journal of Medicinie* 1997; 337: 910–915.

Hyman SE, Arana GW, Rosenbaum, JF. *Handbook of Psychiatric Drug Therapy*. Boston: Little, Brown, 1995.

Kaplan HI, Sadock BJ. *Synopsis of Psychiatry*, 8th ed. Baltimore: Williams & Wilkins, 1997.

Klerman GL, Weissman MM, Rounsaville BJ, Chevron ES. *Interpersonal Psychotherapy of Depression*. New York: Basic Books, 1984.

Langs R. *The Technique of Psychoanalytic Psychotherapy*, Vols. 1 and 2. New York: Jason Aronson, 1974.

Lewis JM. *To Be a Therapist: The Teaching and Learning*. New York: Brunner/ Mazel, 1978.

Lewis M, ed. *A Child and Adolescent Psychiatry Comprehensive Textbook*, 2nd ed. Baltimore: Williams & Wilkins, 1996.

Lifson LE, Simon RI, eds. *The Mental Health Practitioner and the Law: A Comprehensive Textbook*. Cambridge, MA: Harvard University Press, 1998.

Linehan MM. *Cognitive-Behavioral Treatment of Borderline Personality Disorder*. New York: Guilford Press, 1993.

Linehan MM. *Skills Training Manual for Treating Borderline Personality Disorder*. New York: Guilford Press, 1993.

Messner E. *Resilience Enhancement for the Resident Physician*. Durant, OK: Essential Medical Systems, 1993.

Messner E, Groves JE, Schwartz JH, eds. *What Therapists Learn About Themselves & How They Learn It: Autognosis*. Northvale, NJ: Jason Aronson, 1994.

Miller NS. *Principles and Practice of Addictions in Psychiatry*. Philadelphia: W.B. Saunders, 1996.

Miller WR, Rollnick S. *Motivational Interviewing: Preparing People for Change*, 2nd ed. New York: Guilford Press, 2002.

Mitchell SA, Black MJ. *Freud and Beyond: A History of Modern Psychoanalytic Thought*. New York: Basic Books, 1995.

Nemeroff CB, Schatzberg AF. *Recognition and Treatment of Psychiatric Disorders: A Psychopharmacology Handbook for Primary Care*. Washington, DC: American Psychiatric Press, 1999.

Phelan TW. *All about Attention Deficit Disorder*, 2nd ed. Glen Ellyn, IL: Child Management, 2000.

Platt FW, Gordon GH. *Field Guide to the Difficult Patient Interview*. Philadelphia: Lippincott Williams & Wilkins, 1999. (Though written for physicians, much of this book may be useful for nonmedical therapists as well.)

Stern TA, Herman JB, eds. *Psychiatry Update and Board Preparation.* New York: McGraw-Hill, 2000.

Stern TA, Herman JB, Slavin PL, eds. *MGH Guide to Psychiatry in Primary Care.* New York: McGraw-Hll, 1998.

Storr A. *The Art of Psychotherapy.* New York: Routledge Press, 1979.

Waldinger RI. Boundary crossings and boundary violations: Thoughts on navigating a slippery slope. *Harvard Review of Psychiatry* 1994; 2: 225–227.

Acknowledgments

Many individuals helped us bring this book into being.

Our editors at The Guilford Press, Kitty Moore and Jim Nageotte, provided remarkably astute ideas and sustaining encouragement throughout this process. We also want to thank senior production editor Laura Patchkofsky; art director Paul Gordon; marketing director Marian Robinson; and copy editor Jeanne Ford.

We are indebted to Ronald Schouten, MD, JD, Carolyn Wood, JD, and Marilyn McMahon, JD, for their input on psychotherapy issues related to the law and Scott Rauch, MD, for assistance with our neuroscientific questions.

Randy King, MD, PhD, Aimee Bender, and David Bender, MD, were directly helpful to both of us, providing insightful suggestions as the book evolved.

(S. B.): It takes a village to cultivate a professional. I am very grateful for the input, support, and expertise from the accomplished psychiatrists and psychotherapists who supervised me during my training. Their ideas and wisdom provided the guidance I needed. At the University of California, San Francisco: Drs. Jeanne Burns, Mary Margaret McClure, Lynn Ponton, and Chris Wallis. At Harvard, and Massachusetts General Hospital (MGH): Drs. Robert Abernethy, Steve Ablon, Anne Alonso, Eugene Beresin, Joseph Biederman, Jeff Bostic, Barbara Breslau, Susan Brown, Thrassos Calligas, Edwin Cassem, Ginger Chappell, Lee Cohen, Don Condie, Cornelia Cremens, Patricia Doherty, Jim Ellison, David Gastfriend, Edye Geringer, Donald Goff, Paul Hamburg, Patricia Harney, David Henderson, John Herman, David Herzog, Elyce Kearns, Michael Jellinek, Elizabeth Marks, Bruce Masek, John Matthews, Martin Miller, Steve Nickman, Jacqui Olds, Miriam Ornstein, Susan Penava, Patricia Pickett, Mark Pollack, Joseph Schwartz, Ted Stern, Kathy Sanders,

Elizabeth Shapiro-Powers, Judy Teicholz, Jennifer Rathbun, Paula Rauch, Bob Reifsnyder, Jerrold Rosenbaum, Gary Sachs, Larry Selter, Lois Slovik, Tom Spencer, Andrew Stromberg, Tim Wilens, Jonathon Worth, and Janet Wozniak. Marilyn Schwartz, Carolyn Sprich, Alice Curnin, Genevieve Coyle, and Liza Schneiderman provided insight from the social work perspective. The list is long, but it reflects the breadth and depth of the Boston psychiatric community.

My great colleagues enrich my work. I am a better psychiatrist because of Drs. Donna Chen, Deborah Kadish, Julie Newman-Toker, Ruta Nonacs, Alicia Powell, Michael Rater, and Steve Schlozman.

My patients teach me a great deal. I am grateful for the opportunity and privilege to work with them so closely.

My family deserves special mention. My mother has served as an example of an inspired working mother. She bolstered my creativity when I couldn't find it. Karen taught me the power of storytelling and paved the way. Aimee's unrelenting encouragement and courageous example made it possible for me to persevere. And my father, my first mentor in this field, provided me with the inspiration to become a psychiatrist, with gentle and wise oversight all along the way. Last, and so crucial: my husband, Randy. His insight, strength, and character inspire me. I wouldn't be who I am today without his support and love.

Index

325